Innovative Management of Atrial Fibrillation

To my parents Edith and Irving, for their unceasing support and patience
To my wife Susan and our children Emma,
Will, Katie and Ellie – the loves of my life

DS

To my parents Antonio and Tina for their inspiration
To my wife Chiara Hayganoush and our children Giovanni,
Francesco and Alessandro for their love

MAZ

Innovative Management of Atrial Fibrillation

Edited by

David Schwartzman, MD
Associate Professor of Medicine
Director, Atrial Arrhythmia Center, University of Pittsburgh Medical Center

and

Marco A. Zenati, MD
Associate Professor of Surgery
Director, Minimally Invasive Cardiac Surgery, University of Pittsburgh Medical Center

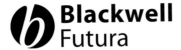 **Blackwell** Futura

First published 2005

ISBN-13: 978-1-4051-2209-2
ISBN-10: 1-4051-2209-9

Library of Congress Cataloging-in-Publication Data
Innovative management of atrial fibrillation / edited by David Schwartzman and Marco Zenati.
     p. ; cm.
   Includes bibliographical references and index.
   ISBN 1-4051-2209-9
   1. Atrial fibrillation–Treatment.
   [DNLM: 1. Atrial Fibrillation–therapy. WG 330 I55 2005]   I. Schwartzman, David, 1959–
II. Zenati, Marco.

RC685.A72I55 2005
616.1′2806–dc22

                                                                                    2004029184

A catalogue record for this title is available from the British Library

Acquisitions: Steve Korn
Development Editor: Vicki Donald
Set in 9.5/12pt Palatino by Graphicraft Limited, Hong Kong
Printed and bound by Replika Press Pvt. Ltd, India

For further information on Blackwell Publishing, visit our website:
www.blackwellcardiology.com

The publisher's policy is to use permanent paper from mills that operate a sustainable forestry
policy, and which has been manufactured from pulp processed using acid-free and elementary
chlorine-free practices. Furthermore, the publisher ensures that the text paper and cover board
used have met acceptable environmental accreditation standards.

Notice: The indications and dosages of all drugs in this book have been recommended in the
medical literature and conform to the practices of the general community. The medications
described do not necessarily have specific approval by the Food and Drug Administration for
use in the diseases and dosages for which they are recommended. The package insert for each
drug should be consulted for use and dosage as approved by the FDA. Because standards for
usage change, it is advisable to keep abreast of revised recommendations, particularly those
concerning new drugs.

Contents

List of Contributors

Willem P. Beukema, MD
Department of Cardiology, Isala Klinieken,
Zwolle, The Netherlands

J. David Burkhardt, MD
Staff Cardiologist, Cleveland Clinic Foundation,
Cleveland, Ohio, USA

J. Kevin Donahue, MD
Assistant Professor of Medicine, Division
of Cardiology, Institute for Molecular
Cardiobiology, Johns Hopkins
University School of Medicine, Baltimore,
Maryland, USA

Joachim R. Ehrlich, MD
Cardiology Fellow, University of Frankfurt,
Frankfurt-am-Main, Germany, Department of
Medicine, Division of Cardiology, Montreal
Heart Institute and University of Montreal,
Montreal, Quebec, Canada

Arif Elvan, MD, PhD
Department of Cardiology, Isala Klinieken,
Zwolle, The Netherlands

Heather Fraser, MD
Post-Doctoral, Institute for Molecular
Cardiobiology, Johns Hopkins
University School of Medicine,
Baltimore, Maryland, USA

A. Marc Gillinov, MD
Staff Surgeon, Department of Thoracic and
Cardiovascular Surgery, Surgical Director,
Center for Atrial Fibrillation, Cleveland Clinic
Foundation, Cleveland, Ohio, USA

Michel Haissaguerre, MD
Professor, Department of Cardiology,
Haut-Leveque Hospital, University of
Bordeaux, Bordeaux, France

Alan H. Heldman, MD
Associate Professor of Medicine, Institute for
Molecular Cardiobiology, Johns Hopkins
University School of Medicine, Baltimore,
Maryland, USA

Douglas Hettrick, PhD
Senior Principal Scientist, Medtronic Inc.,
Minneapolis, Minnesota, USA

Pierre Jais, MD
Staff Cardiologist, Department of Cardiology,
Haut-Leveque Hospital, University of Bordeaux,
Bordeaux, France

Jonathan M. Kalman, MBBS, PhD
Professor of Medicine, Department of Cardiology,
Royal Melbourne Hospital and Department of
Medicine, University of Melbourne, Melbourne,
Australia

Randall Lee, MD, PhD
Associate Professor of Medicine, Division of
Cardiology, Department of Medicine, University
of California San Francisco, San Francisco,
California, USA

Barry London, MD, PhD
Associate Professor of Medicine, Chief, Division
of Cardiology, and Director, Cardiovascular
Institute, University of Pittsburgh Medical Center,
Pittsburgh, Pennsylvania, USA

Patrick M. McCarthy, MD
Surgical Director, George M. and Linda H.
Kaufman Center for Heart Failure, The Center for
Atrial Fibrillation, Cleveland Clinic Foundation,
Cleveland, Ohio, USA

Amy McDonald, BS
Research Tech II, Department of Medicine,
Cardiovascular, Institute for Molecular
Cardiobiology, Johns Hopkins University School
of Medicine, Baltimore, Maryland, USA

Julie M. Miller, MD
Assistant Professor of Medicine, Institute for
Molecular Cardiobiology, Johns Hopkins
University School of Medicine, Baltimore,
Maryland, USA

Anand R. Ramdat Misier, MD, PhD
Department of Cardiology, Isala Klinieken,
Zwolle, The Netherlands

Joseph B. Morton, MBBS
Doctoral Research Fellow, Department of Cardiology, Royal Melbourne Hospital and Department of Medicine, University of Melbourne, Melbourne, Australia

Stanley Nattel, MD
Professor of Medicine, Paul-David Chair in Cardiovascular Electrophysiology, Department of Medicine, Division of Cardiology, Montreal Heart Institute, Montreal, Quebec, Canada

Paul S. Pagel, MD, PhD
Director, Cardiac Anesthesia, Professor of Anesthesiology, Medical College of Wisconsin, Milwaukee, Wisconsin, USA

Jeffrey J. Rade, MD
Assistant Professor of Medicine, Institute for Molecular Cardiobiology, Johns Hopkins University School of Medicine, Baltimore, Maryland, USA

Samir Saba, MD
Division of Cardiac Electrophysiology, University of Pittsburgh, Cardiovascular Institute, University of Pittsburgh Medical Center, Pittsburgh, Pennsylvania, USA

Prashanthan Sanders, MBBS
Doctoral Research Fellow, Department of Cardiology, Royal Melbourne Hospital and Department of Medicine, University of Melbourne, Melbourne, Australia

David Schwartzman, MD
Associate Professor of Medicine, Presbyterian University Hospital, 200 Lothrop Street, Room B535, Pittsburgh, Pennsylvania, USA

Dipen Shah, MD
Médecin Adjoint, Division of Cardiology, Electrophysiology, Hôpital Cantonal de Genève, Geneva, Switzerland

Vladimir Shusterman, MD, PhD
Director, Noninvasive Laboratories, Cardiovascular Institute, University of Pittsburgh, Pittsburgh, Pennsylvania, USA

Hauw T. Sie, MD
Department of Cardiothoracic Surgery, Isala Klinieken, Zwolle, The Netherlands

Paul B. Sparks, MBBS, PhD
Cardiologist, Department of Cardiology, Royal Melbourne Hospital, Melbourne, Australia

Hung-Fat Tse, MD
Associate Professor, Department of Medicine, University of Hong Kong, Queen Mary Hospital, Hong Kong

Michael Ujhelyi, PharmD
Senior Principal Scientist, Medtronic Inc., Minneapolis, Minnesota, USA

Bruce L. Wilkoff, MD
Director, Cardiac Pacing and Tachyarrhythmia Devices, Cleveland Clinic Foundation, Cleveland, Ohio, USA

Marco A. Zenati, MD
Associate Professor of Surgery, University of Pittsburgh Medical Center/Presbyterian University Hospital, Division of Cardiothoracic Surgery, Pittsburgh, Pennsylvania, USA

Preface

[Innovation] may mean simply the realization that there is no particular virtue in doing things the way that they have always been done

Rudolph Flesch

Atrial fibrillation (AF) is associated with an impressive burden [1]. Independent of comorbidity, it is associated with a substantial increase in the risk of death. It is associated with left ventricular systolic dysfunction and congestive heart failure. AF is causal of embolic cerebrovascular accident. The proportion of cerebrovascular accident attributable to AF increases with age; it is the most common etiology in the elderly. AF is associated with dementia. Although the nature of this relationship is not clear, some data suggest that recurrent subclinical cerebral embolic events may play a role [2]. AF is associated with a marked diminishment in patient-perceived life quality and a high rate of utilization of health-care resources. These factors play into a large and multi-faceted economic burden, extending beyond the affected individual to involve their families, health-care providers and governments.

The incidence and prevalence of AF are rising. Although presently estimated at 2–3 million persons (US), the prevalence is expected to exceed 5 million by the year 2010, indicative of an epidemic [3]. Given its mechanistic link to obesity and hypertension, our expectation is that the incidence will continue to increase in decades to come. It is crucial to understand that AF occurs commonly in the setting of otherwise healthy aging.

Why is innovation necessary?

AF provides a useful window to the limitations of cardiovascular disease prevention and management as it is presently practised. Although a causal association between AF and cerebrovascular events is not disputed, the disease is underdiagnosed and preventative strategies are underutilized. In addition, although clearly a biomarker for subsequent cardiovascular morbidity and mortality, a diagnosis of AF does not in routine practice evoke more aggressive attempts at prevention, and it is not used effectively as a motivational tool. In terms of management, studies to date have not demonstrated the superiority of atrial rhythm over ventricular rate control. However, a fair comparison remains elusive because of the poor efficacy and tolerability of atrial rhythm control strategies. In this regard, it remains unclear as to what pathophysiological elements of AF underlie morbidity, and in what relative proportions.

How should we proceed?

We believe that the first order of business should involve increasing public and practitioner awareness of AF and increasing the proportion of patients appropriately managed with warfarin. In our institution, public and professional seminars are held regularly. Print and video media outlets are accessed regularly. Electrophysiologist follow-up after emergency department visits for atrial tachyarrhythmia is automated. Hospital care pathways specific for AF have been devised. A central facility for rhythm monitoring has been established, with easy access for clinicians who wish to pursue symptoms. A central facility for warfarin management staffed by pharmacists has been established, at no cost to the patient or the referring physician.

For individual patients with AF, it is our thesis that the diagnosis should evoke an aggressive, sustained effort to prevent downstream *all-cause* cardiovascular morbidity and mortality. It has been our experience that common accompaniments of AF are hypertension, obesity, sedentary lifestyle, dyslipidemia and 'pathopsychology'. The latter entity contains elements of anxiety and depression. We take a multidisciplinary approach, involving longitudinal involvement of nurse-educator, nutritionist, exercise physiologist and psychologist. We place equal emphasis on the concept that AF is a warning of worse things to come (cerebrovascular accident, myocardial infarction) as we do on its treatment.

The development of rate and rhythm control therapies for AF will depend in part on clarification of what is necessary. Although restitution and maintenance of sinus rhythm is desirable in a vacuum, difficulty in achieving this goal will temper development if it cannot be demonstrated to alter outcome. For example, that ventricular rate control is an important element of necessary management has been demonstrated, but the additive value of uniform atrial electrical activation is clear. Nevertheless, there is presently an intense multidisciplinary effort to achieve rhythm control. Given the limitations of pharmacotherapy for this purpose, innovative non-pharmacological therapies have attracted great interest. Modalities which are currently being assessed include atrial ablation, pacing and defibrillation. These efforts clearly have promise but are as yet immature. New modalities have also been proposed based on burgeoning knowledge in areas such as tissue engineering and molecular cardiology. In addition, therapies to achieve rate control and reduce AF-attributable embolic risk are also under development.

Our goal for this book is to provide a snapshot of a rapidly moving target: the non-pharmacological management of patients with AF. We have asked a group of prominent authors with significant experience and insight to summarize their work and to place it in the context of future development. We have also included authors whose work has heretofore not been applied to AF management but for which it has significant promise. We are indebted to these authors for their contributions.

DS
MAZ

Acknowledgements

The dedication to this project of Lorri Courtright is gratefully recognized.

References

1 Fuster V, Ryden LE, Asinger RW *et al.* ACC/AHA/ESC guidelines for the management of patients with atrial fibrillation: executive summary. *J Am Coll Cardiol* 2001; **38**: 1231–66.

2 Tinkler K, Cullinane M, Kaposzta Z *et al.* Asymptomatic embolization in non-valvular atrial fibrillation and its relationship to anticoagulation therapy. *Eur J Ultrasound* 2002; **15**: 21–7.

3 Go AS, Hylek EM, Phillips KA *et al.* P Prevalence of diagnosed atrial fibrillation in adults: national implications for rhythm management and stroke prevention: the AnTicoagulation and Risk Factors in Atrial Fibrillation (ATRIA) Study. *JAMA* 2001; **285**: 2370–5.

PART I

On the Atrial Substrate

CHAPTER 1

Electrophysiological Basis of Atrial Fibrillation

Joachim R. Ehrlich, Stanley Nattel

This chapter deals with the individual structural, functional and ionic bases of atrial fibrillation (AF) under various clinical conditions. We focus on factors that may play a role in setting up a favorable milieu for the arrhythmia and determinants of AF initiation. In addition, factors maintaining AF and possible therapeutic interventions will be discussed. In the first part of this chapter, we will outline mechanisms initiating AF. We will discuss localization of clinical triggers and the changes in atrial electrophysiology that occur in disease states that are commonly associated with an increased incidence of paroxysmal or persistent AF. Clinical conditions like coronary artery disease, congestive heart failure (CHF) and vagally mediated AF will be examined with consideration given to how these change atrial electrophysiology to lead to initiation and maintenance of AF. The second part of the chapter summarizes the structural and functional changes that promote the maintenance of AF by virtue of atrial tachycardia (AT)-induced remodeling once AF has occurred. In the third part, specific implications for therapeutic interventions are considered. AF exists in varying forms that range from spontaneously terminating (paroxysmal) forms to forms that are lasting but are possible to terminate (persistent) and even impossible to terminate (permanent) [1]. The relative roles of triggers and substrates in these forms are shown schematically in Fig. 1.1.

Atrial fibrillation initiation

Triggers

Spontaneous AF is usually initiated by atrial premature complexes (APCs) that couple with a short interval to the preceding beat [2]. Often, APCs initiate a short run of regular AT that precedes the onset of AF. Unlike the situation in ventricular tachycardia or torsade de pointes, no specific activation sequence (e.g. long–short) is usually observed at the onset of AF [3]. Although clinical AF may begin apparently *de novo*, a great number of episodes seen clinically are started by a single APC [4]. This behavior can be reproduced experimentally. When animals are subjected to rapid atrial pacing, increased vulnerability to AF induction by single premature stimuli appears, whereas little or no AF can be induced by APCs in non-paced animals. [5]. Thus, although APCs are capable

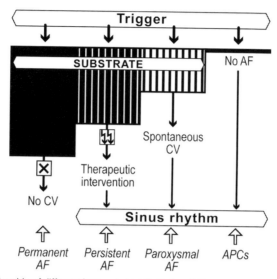

Fig. 1.1 The relationship of different forms of atrial fibrillation (AF) encountered in clinical practice to the underlying substrate. Triggers are required for initiation of atrial re-entry. Where a significant re-entrant substrate is lacking, triggers will remain isolated atrial premature complexes (APCs) without further consequence. In paroxysmal AF, the substrate allows AF initiation but is insufficient for AF persistence. In persistent AF, the substrate allows stable AF, but effective AF termination is still possible. If the substrate progresses, AF may become permanent and no longer amenable to cardioversion. CV = cardioversion; SR = sinus rhythm.

of initiating AF they will not always do so; they need a susceptible substrate. Consequently, it is crucial to understand the substrate that renders the atria susceptible to AF initiation by individual triggers and then to put trigger and substrate into context in each clinical setting [6].

APCs may initiate AF from nearly anywhere within the atria. However, certain areas are particularly prone to producing arrhythmogenic APCs: the pulmonary veins (PVs) [7], superior vena cava (SVC), [4, 8], crista terminalis, right atrioventricular junction and superior left atrium (LA) [9] have all been demonstrated to give rise to AF-triggering APCs. Sites of demonstrated trigger activity are illustrated in Fig. 1.2.

Endocardial mapping studies by Saksena *et al.* demonstrated various characteristics of the onset of spontaneous AF [2, 9]. These investigators found that the earliest atrial activation during initiation of spontaneous AF was close to the site of spontaneous APCs within LA and the right atrium (RA) observed during electrophysiological study. Consistent with data obtained by electrogram recording in the 1970s [10], a high degree of organization in the electrograms was generally present before AF became sustained. The authors attributed this to a possible initial spiral-wave/rotor mechanism triggering AF by generation of multiple daughter wavelets. LA onset of AF was more common among patients without heart disease, whereas patients with hyper-

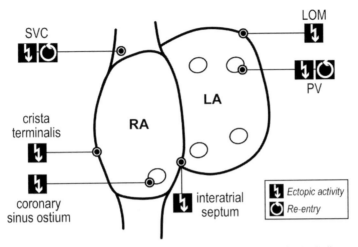

Fig. 1.2 Localization of structures in human atria involved in AF initiation. Circles indicate preferential re-entry, flashes indicate focal ectopic activity. LOM = ligament of Marshall; PV = pulmonary vein; SVC = superior vena cava.

tension or coronary artery disease had more frequent initiation from the RA. Overall, the authors demonstrated significant heterogeneity in onset regions, arguing against a single left or RA trigger location for AF [9]. When AF was induced by programmed RA stimulation, heterogeneity of conduction delay was present, with maxima at the coronary sinus ostium, the His bundle region and the interatrial septum. At these locations fragmented potentials (including double potentials) were often seen, suggesting the existence of conduction block possibly contributing to AF initiation and indicating the potential import-ance of substrate factors [2]. Other investigators have also noted RA focal AF sources in a small proportion of patients [11]. The APCs involved originated primarily in the coronary sinus ostium and the crista terminalis. Ablation of these foci cured AF.

The myocardial sleeves of PVs are a particularly important locus of AF initiation. PV foci trigger a high percentage of clinical AF episodes in patients without structural heart disease [7, 12]. Overall, the superior PVs (with longer myocardial sleeves) are more involved in triggering AF than inferior ones, but foci have been demonstrated in all PV locations. Some observers have reported a relationship between the length of PV sleeves and the sites of APCs causing AF, with foci tending to be located distally (2–4 cm beyond the PV–LA junction) [13]. However, a recent study pointed to the importance of the proximal parts of the PVs [4]. The mechanism leading to PV ectopic activity appears to be non-re-entrant, as the arrhythmia could not be induced by programmed stimulation [7]. Some experimental studies have shown abnormal automaticity and triggered activity in PV preparations, suggesting that PVs are a virtual Pandora's box of arrhythmogenesis, even in healthy canine tissue [14]. However, other workers were unable to demonstrate triggered activity or spontaneous depolarizations in normal canine PVs [15]. The architecture of the PVs may facilitate micro-re-entry by virtue of structural complexities, leading to heterogeneous impulse propagation with marked slowing at regions of directional discontinuity [15]. Optical mapping suggests that re-entry may be the predominant arrhythmia mechanism within normal PV myocardium [16].

Just as the PV myocardium is connected to the LA, the SVC is partially covered by sleeves of myocardium that are in continuity with the RA. Tsai *et al.* described eight patients with spontaneous AF initiated by a burst of rapid ectopic beats originating ~2 cm distally to the junction between SVC and RA [8]. During 9 months following successful ablation of the SVC foci, all patients remained free of AF relapse. Two patients manifested sinus rhythm after ablation despite persistent fibrillatory activity inside the SVC. Other investigators reported findings in a patient with longstanding AF and atrial flutter. During electrophysiological study, a regular re-entrant tachycardia in the SVC with a cycle length of 230 ms was documented, which may have played a role triggering AF [17]. In keeping with these findings, 17 patients with paroxysmal AF after PV ablation were subsequently successfully treated with radiofrequency ablation of connections between the SVC and the RA [18].

Other structures within the LA may also exhibit arrhythmogenic activity. The ligament of Marshall (LOM) was first noted to be a focal source of adrenergically sensitive automatic activity in experimental studies on dogs [19]. Isoproterenol infusion led to rapidly firing LOM foci in tissues of healthy dogs as well as dogs subjected to rapid atrial pacing. Only rapidly paced dogs developed AF. A similar role in AF initiation was suggested for cases of human AF, with ablation of LOM potentials eliminating the arrhythmia [20]. The possible role of the LOM as a triggering site in adrenergically mediated AF is emphasized by studies demonstrating a high concentration of sympathetic nerve fibers in human LOM [21].

The specific cellular mechanisms underlying the formation of special clinical triggering regions are poorly understood. Triggered activity may result from delayed or early afterdepolarizations. Diastolic cellular depolarization, primarily through electrogenic Na^+/Ca^{2+} exchange in the presence of intracellular Ca^{2+} overload, underlie delayed afterdepolarizations. Reactivation of L-type calcium channels during prolonged action potentials may underlie early afterdepolarizations. Abnormal automaticity may also be relevant in the genesis of AF, if phase 4 depolarization is accelerated, causing threshold to be reached prematurely and APCs to be initiated. Focal cellular activity that could trigger AF has been reported in PV myocytes, even from healthy canine hearts [14, 22]. However, other laboratories were unable to demonstrate any spontaneous activity under control conditions [15]. Data on SVC automaticity also remain rudimentary [23]. PV effective refractory periods (RPs) are shorter in patients with AF [24], perhaps contributing to their arrhythmogenic properties. Potential mechanisms of PV activity that have been reported are provided in Table 1.1.

Table 1.1 Potential mechanisms of pulmonary vein activity

Reference	Species	Key findings	Spontaneous APs
Cheung (1981)[93]	guinea-pig	– digitalis-induced tachycardia – slow automaticity	+
Chen et al. (2001)[14]	dog	– rapid spontaneous depolarization – triggered activity	+
Chen et al. (2002)[94]	rabbit	– rapid spontaneous depolarization – triggered activity	+
Hocini et al. (2002)[15]	dog	– anatomic structure in favor of re-entry – slow conduction	–
Arora et al. (2003)[16]	dog	– re-entry with single extra-stimulus – slow focal activity after isoproterenol	–
Luk et al. (2003)[95]	dog	– homogeneous distribution of fast response APs in PVs	–

Substrate

Although premature beat triggers are important in AF initiation, the ability of single extrastimuli to initiate atrial re-entry and AF depends on the atrial substrate. Furthermore, the likelihood that AF will be sustained once initiated is very substrate-dependent [25]. The ability to maintain re-entrant arrhythmias is believed to depend on the wavelength (distance traveled by an impulse during the RP), which is given by the product of conduction velocity and RP. The wavelength gives the size of the shortest circuit that can maintain re-entry and determines the size of functional re-entrant circuits. The larger the wavelength, the fewer circuits a given atrium can accommodate and the less likely AF is to be sustained. An ideal substrate for re-entry thus would involve slowing of impulse propagation (e.g. due to decreased Na^+ current, or passive conduction abnormalities like tissue fibrosis or abnormal cell-connecting connexin proteins) and would also shorten the RP (by decreasing action potential duration (APD), which is the most important cellular determinant of the RP). Furthermore, RP heterogeneity is also important in promoting re-entry [5, 26]. Atrial regions known to play a prominent role in re-entry are shown in Fig. 1.2.

Besides triggering the arrhythmia, PVs may be an important part of the environment for the maintenance of AF. They play an important role in persistent AF, albeit not as critical as their role in triggering arrhythmia in paroxysmal AF without structural heart disease. Ablation/isolation of PV myocardial sleeves suppresses AF in from ~30% [12] to ~70% [27] of patients with persistent AF, although in the latter study the extensive LA ablation makes it difficult to be sure that benefit was exclusively due to PV elimination. PV muscle fascicles within the myocardial sleeves display a great degree of decremental conduction and significant heterogeneity in conduction properties and refractoriness [28]. Together with their complex anatomical structure [15], PVs are a favorable site for re-entrant arrhythmias [16]. Fibrillatory activation may be maintained and re-initiated in isolated PVs after electrophysiological disconnection from the LA [29]. PVs may thus represent both triggers for AF initiation and a key part of the substrate for AF maintenance.

Tissue stretch can promote AF by inducing triggered activity or by affecting atrial refractory properties. In clinical conditions like hypertension, mitral stenosis and CHF, which lead to increased atrial pressure or volume overload and are classically associated with AF, these mechanisms may contribute to the AF substrate. Whereas chronic stretch is present in these clinical conditions, acute stretch may occur with ruptured chordae tendineae, extensive acute myocardial infarction or hypertensive crisis. Acute atrial stretch leads to shortening of APD and RP, facilitating initiation and maintenance of AF [30, 31]. However, there is controversy about the changes in action potential morphology and RP induced by atrial stretch (summarized by Bosch and Nattel [32]). In isolated rabbit hearts, increased atrial filling pressure is associated with increased inducibility of AF and shortening of refractoriness [31]. Other investigators found prolongation of atrial APD and RP rather than shortening in dogs, and results in humans are variable [30]. Valvuloplasty for congenital pulmonary stenosis decreases APD of right ventricular monophasic action potentials [33]. A possible cellular basis for increased vulnerability to AF is the activation of stretch-activated channels (SACs). These non-specific cationic SACs (permeant to Ca^{2+}, Na^+ and K^+) enhance automaticity by depolarizing cells. Inhibition of SACs antagonizes the AF-promoting effect of acute stretch, while the stretch-induced shortening of the RP remains unaffected [34]. The effects of chronic stretch have been studied in humans during mitral valve commissurotomy [35]. Chronically increased atrial pressure leads to intra-atrial conduction slowing, shortened RP and increased vulnerability to AF, which is at least partly reversible. AF vulnerability and the heterogeneity of conduction delay are significantly correlated with LA pressure. In patients with a history of AF, RP heterogeneity was increased before and normalized after commissurotomy, whereas no increased heterogeneity was present among sinus-rhythm patients. Chronic stretch may also be associated with electrical remodeling. Cells isolated from dilated human atria have markedly shortened APDs compared with cells from non-dilated atria and show decreased calcium current, which could account for the shorter APD [36].

AF complicates 6–26% of cases of acute myocardial infarction [37, 38], although the incidence is declining [39]. Patients with AF within 24 hours after myocardial infarction have a significantly greater incidence of occlusion of the proximal right coronary artery (with increased RA pressure) compared with patients in sinus rhythm [40]. Similarly, patients with right ventricular myocardial infarction have a higher incidence of APCs that could trigger AF [41]. The precise mechanisms of AF promotion by acute infarction are unclear. One study suggested that infarct-related pericarditis may increase the risk of AF [42]. Atrial stretch associated with acute LV dysfunction is another potential contributor. Increased atrial pressure has been linked to greater susceptibility to atrial arrhythmias in a rat infarction model [43]. Acute atrial ischemia creates a substrate for re-entrant AF in association with marked conduction slowing in the ischemic zone [44]. Thus, atrial ischemia provides a substrate for AF by mechanisms similar to those well-demonstrated to promote ventricular fibrillation in acute ventricular ischemia, including heterogeneous APD changes and marked conduction slowing [45].

CHF and AF are the 'emerging epidemics of cardiovascular disease' [46] and CHF is a very important cause of clinical AF. AF is present in 40–50% of patients with NYHA functional class IV compared with ~10% in patients with NYHA class II [47]. Besides atrial stretch associated with increased ventricular filling pressures and activation of neurohumoral pathways, CHF alters atrial tissue composition and produces electrical remodeling. Experimental CHF promotes AF, causing interstitial fibrosis and localized conduction abnormalities, without affecting global conduction, RP or RP heterogeneity [48]. CHF-related conduction abnormalities produce a substrate for AF due to macro-re-entry with fibrillatory conduction [49]. At the ionic level, the slow component of the delayed rectifier current (I_{Ks}), L-type calcium current ($I_{Ca,L}$) and transient outward current (I_{to}) are reduced [50]. Although this balanced change in inward and outward currents leaves APD largely unaffected, the electrogenic Na^+/Ca^{2+} exchanger is upregulated, potentially promoting delayed afterdepolarizations which could trigger atrial arrhythmias. Thus, CHF may induce both a favorable substrate and potential triggers.

Vagally mediated AF is a well-described clinical entity affecting mostly patients without structural heart disease. Some patients may have a specific bradycardic threshold below which they experience AF onset and may even be able to prevent this onset by physical exercise. Acetylcholine heterogeneously shortens the atrial RP without affecting conduction velocity. At the onset of vagal AF, the local atrial response is extremely rapid (rates of up to 900/min have been reported) [51]. In isolated canine RA the underlying arrhythmic mechanism appeared to be a relatively stable re-entrant circuit giving rise to fibrillatory excitation [52]. Computer simulation suggests that vagal AF might result from acetylcholine-induced stabilization of a spiral wave with complex conduction through heterogeneously responding tissue [53]. At the cellular level, APD is abbreviated by the activation of acetylcholine-induced inward rectifier K^+ current ($I_{K,ACh}$), which accelerates repolarization. Circadian patterns of AF onset show an influence of the autonomous nervous system. Paroxysmal AF onset occurs during the daytime in elderly patients with underlying heart disease, implying a predominant role of sympathetic tone [54]. A recent study applying frequency-domain analysis of heart-rate variability suggested a primary increase in adrenergic tone followed by an abrupt shift toward vagal predominance, leading to AF initiation [55].

Thyrotoxicosis is an important risk factor for AF. Adrenergic nervous system hyperactivity may play an important role in mediating the effects of elevated thyroid hormones on the heart. Hyperthyroidism reduces atrial APD and RP. Experimental data regarding ionic mechanisms are variable and sometimes contradictory. Work in guinea-pigs showed upregulation of slow delayed rectifier potassium current (I_{Ks}) and calcium current ($I_{Ca,L}$) [56], whereas mRNA levels encoding the underlying subunits were unaffected. These results could explain APD shortening on the basis of increased I_{Ks}. Micro-array gene analysis of adult mouse ventricular myocytes showed upregulation of the alpha- and beta-subunits underlying I_{Ks} (KCNQ1 and KCNE1) in hypothyroidism, and a converse downregulation in hyperthyroidism [57]. Unlike in guinea-pig myocytes, KCNQ1 and KCNE1 do not contribute significantly to repolarization in the mouse. Thus, the functional relevance of the changes observed in mice as well as the cellular mechanism by which thyrotoxicosis forms a substrate for AF remain to be determined.

Atrial fibrillation sustenance

The following section concisely focuses on changes in atrial electrophysiology and structure that facilitate AF maintenance. Many of the results summarized in this section were obtained from studies carried out in animals. Wherever possible, experimental findings will be correlated with results from studies involving human patients. For further detailed information we refer to recent reviews [25, 32, 58, 59].

Once AF occurs, the atria accommodate to the rapid activation rate by downregulating I_{Ca}, which protects the cell from Ca^{2+} overload but makes it easier for AF to become sustained. This electrical remodeling results from sustained rapid atrial activation, independent of the underlying mechanism. Since the first description by Wijffels *et al.*, AF-induced changes in atrial electrophysiology have been systematically examined in animal models and humans [60]. AF remodeling leads to shorter atrial RP with increased RP heterogeneity and reduced RP rate adaptation. RP particularly decreases at slow heart rates, increasing vulnerability to ectopic beats. RP abbreviation and the AF-promoting effect of AT/AF have been observed in humans as key features of electrical remodeling [58]. Longstanding AF may additionally reduce conduction velocity, by decreasing sodium current (I_{Na}) or causing spatially heterogeneous changes in connexin expression [59]. These features – shortened RP and reduced conduction velocity – decrease wavelength and make sustained re-entrant activation via multiple wavelet re-entry more likely. In dogs, AT decreases RP by reducing APD via downregulation of $I_{Ca,L}$ [61]. Similarly, a prominent reduction of $I_{Ca,L}$ occurs in human AF [62]. Along with Ca^{2+} current, the transient outward potassium current (I_{to}) is also down-regulated by AT. Intracellular calcium-homeostasis is altered and Ca^{2+} overload may jeopardize cell vitality [63]. Slower and smaller Ca^{2+} transients caused by sustained rapid atrial rates decrease atrial myocyte contractility [64] and underlie the atrial contractile dysfunction ('atrial stunning') observed in clinical AF. Reduced membrane currents are associated with reduced levels of corresponding ion-channel mRNA [65]. Other repolarizing currents (I_{Ks}, I_{Kr}, I_{K1}) remain unchanged during ionic remodeling secondary to AT. In the presence of a CHF-induced substrate for sustained AF, the effects of AT on RP are less prominent, and AF promotion is less pronounced compared with AT effects in normal hearts [66].

Abnormal electrical coupling between cardiomyocytes may contribute to disturbed impulse propagation in diseased myocardial tissue. Connexins are gap-junction hemichannel proteins responsible for conduction of electrical impulses between neighboring cells. In the mammalian heart, connexins 37, 40, 43, 45, 46 and 50 (numbers indicate molecular weight in kDa) are present. Connexin 43 is predominant in cardiac tissue and connexin 40 seems to be specifically localized in atria. There is dispute about the relevance of changes in connexins in AT remodeling. Whereas atrial connexin 43 content remains unaffected during long-lasting AT in goats, reduction and spatial disorganization of connexin 40 expression can be observed [67]. These changes are correlated with increased inducibility and stability of AF without detectable conduction slowing. On the other hand, AF is associated with connexin 43 upregulation in dogs [68].

Contractile dysfunction induced by AF has been recognized for over 30 years. After cardioversion to sinus rhythm, the A-wave in the LA pressure curve disappears and months elapse before atrial contraction fully recovers [69]. Sustained AT similarly leads to contractile dysfunction of isolated cardiomyocytes, along with reduced intracellular Ca^{2+} transients [64]. As L-type calcium current determines Ca^{2+} content and release from the sarcoplasmic reticulum, downregulation of $I_{Ca,L}$ is likely to be at least partially responsible for contractile dysfunction. In CHF, the number of viable myocytes is decreased and replacement of space formerly occupied by myocytes with fibrotic tissue occurs. This increase in fibrotic tissue may lead to increased anisotropy of impulse conduction and localized conduction abnormalities that stabilize re-entry [48].

Implications for therapy

Specific therapeutic targets may be deduced from these insights into triggers and substrates [59]. Ablation approaches are effective for suppression of initiation, whereas pharmacological and surgical approaches play a central role in controlling sustenance. The fact that AF is often preceded by an episode of regular AT (as outlined above) may explain the efficacy of antitachycardiac pacing algorithms to suppress AF [70].

Initiation

Technical aspects of atrial ablation are discussed elsewhere in this book. Ablation of myocardium investing the pulmonary veins is highly effective in eliminating AF triggers, and may also be important in attacking the AF substrate. Segmental isolation of PVs where the myocardial sleeve is thickest is sufficient to suppress the arrhythmia [71]. Even patients with longstanding AF due to mitral valve disease can be effectively treated with PV ablation. The more PVs in a single patient are isolated the smaller becomes AF inducibility [72]. In a similar fashion, ablation of other arrhythmogenic sites within the RA or LA (SVC, LOM) has been shown to be a feasible and efficient therapeutic approach.

Sustenance

Verapamil attenuates changes in contractility and electrophysiological properties during short-term AT-remodeling in animal studies and human patients [59]. Changes in longstanding AF are not reversed by L-type calcium channel blockers [73], probably because different mechanisms (like transcriptional downregulation) underlie long-term remodeling, as opposed to the functional changes (ion-channel inactivation) involved in short-term remodeling. The T-type channel blocker mibefradil suppresses the development of AT-remodeling [74]. The effects of mibefradil contrast with those of the L-type I_{Ca} blocker diltiazem, with no efficacy against 1-week AT-remodeling [75]. The timing of drug application may be important, as application of verapamil 1 week before AT onset may prevent development of an AT substrate [76]. The mechanism of mibefradil prevention of electrical remodeling remains unclear. Although T-type channel blockade may be important, mibefradil has other effects that could participate. Mibefradil is unavailable for clinical use because of deleterious side effects due to drug interactions based on cytochrome P450 inhibition. Some studies have indicated a beneficial effect of angiotensin-converting enzyme (ACE) inhibitors or angiotensin II receptor antagonists in preventing remodeling induced by rapid atrial pacing [77]. Na+/H+ exchanger blockers have shown promising results for short-term remodeling [78]. However, during long-term remodeling both approaches have yielded negative results [79].

Since it is hard to predict when AF will occur, the physician is usually faced with reversing the substrate that developed during persistent AF. After termination of AF, AT-remodeling reverses with a time course of days to weeks [80, 81]. Prevention of AF relapse after cardioversion through prolongation of repolarization with class IA or III agents allows reversal of remodeling to occur spontaneously, reducing the risk of re-initiation. Despite normalization of electrophysiological parameters, increased vulnerability to AF may persist [82]. Amiodarone reverses electrical remodeling in experimental animals [83], potentially contributing to its antiarrhythmic efficacy.

Treatments targeting atrial stretch, including inhibitors of SACs and agents improving hemodynamics, may eventually prove useful. Interesting results point towards protective effects of Gs-Mtx-4, a spider venom peptide that selectively inhibits SACs and suppresses stretch-related AF [34]. Verapamil has also been shown to be of some benefit in preventing shortening of the atrial RP in the setting of stretch and rapid activation [84].

As CHF produces a specific atrial substrate that promotes the occurrence and maintenance of AF, this may have the potential for specific therapeutic approaches. For example, interventions to prevent atrial fibrosis may prevent the AF substrate from developing. Enalapril reduces the AF-promoting effect of experimental CHF, probably by interfering with angiotensin II-related intracellular signal transduction mechanisms [85]. It also reduces atrial enlargement and improves hemodynamics, while reducing the duration of induced AF [86]. Since CHF-induced atrial fibrosis appears irreversible [87], early intervention may be important in prevention. The atrial ionic remodeling that occurs in CHF (specifically downregulation of I_{Ks} and I_{K1}) makes repolarization more dependent on the rapid component I_{Kr} [50]. This may explain the effectiveness of dofetilide (a selective I_{Kr} inhibitor) for AF termination in the setting of experimental CHF compared with tachycardia-induced atrial remodeling [88]. In the DIAMOND-CHF trial, treatment with dofetilide was safe and efficacious in the termination of AF and the prevention of recurrence in patients with CHF [89]. In clinical settings, clear-cut differentiation between CHF substrate, atrial stretch and diseases that lead to CHF, such as coronary artery disease, are not so easily made. However, the TRACE study demonstrated that ACE inhibitors prevent AF in patients with reduced left ventricular function following myocardial infarction [90].

The pharmacological treatment of AF is limited by unsatisfactory recurrence rates, and focal ablation may only work in selected patients. The surgical Maze creates lines of block that prevent re-entry and AF. The overall success rate in curing AF has been greater than 95% [91]. The Maze-III procedure (in use since 1992) isolates the PVs, creates linear lesions in the LA and RA and reduces atrial tissue mass by amputating both appendages. It is the most effective therapy presently available for treating medically refractory AF. The major shortcoming of the surgical Maze is the invasiveness of the technique and it is clear that only a tiny percentage of patients with AF are candidates for the open-heart Maze procedure. Catheter-based Maze techniques involving linear ablation lesions are being developed, but are still very much experimental. Another approach combines a minimally invasive surgical technique with intraoperative radiofrequency catheter ablation [92].

Conclusions

The factors important in the initiation and maintenance of AF need to be understood, as individual substrates require different treatment strategies. As more evidence is obtained about AF in different settings, the picture becomes more complex than expected. An appreciation of this complexity may ultimately allow individually targeted AF treatment, although much work remains to be done before mechanism-targeted therapy can become a practical reality.

References

1 Sopher SM, Camm AJ. Atrial fibrillation: maintenance of sinus rhythm versus rate control. *Am J Cardiol* 1996; **77**: 24A–37A.
2 Saksena S, Giorgberidze I, Mehra R *et al.* Electrophysiology and endocardial mapping of induced atrial fibrillation in patients with spontaneous atrial fibrillation. *Am J Cardiol* 1999; **83**: 187–93.

3 Hnatkova K, Waktare JE, Murgatroyd FD, Guo X, Baiyan X, Camm AJ, Malik M. Analysis of the cardiac rhythm preceding episodes of paroxysmal atrial fibrillation. *Am Heart J* 1998; **135**: 1010–19.

4 Lu TM, Tai CT, Hsieh MH *et al*. Electrophysiologic characteristics in initiation of paroxysmal atrial fibrillation from a focal area. *J Am Coll Cardiol* 2001; **37**: 1658–64.

5 Fareh S, Villemaire C, Nattel S. Importance of refractoriness heterogeneity in the enhanced vulnerability to atrial fibrillation induction caused by tachycardia-induced electrical remodeling. *Circulation* 1998; **98**: 2202–9.

6 Wijffels MC, Kirchhof CJ, Dorland R, Power J, Allessie MA. Electrical remodeling due to atrial fibrillation in chronically instrumented conscious goats: roles of neurohumoral changes, ischemia, atrial stretch, and high rate of electrical activation. *Circulation* 1997; **96**: 3710–20.

7 Haissaguerre M, Jais P, Shah DC *et al*. Spontaneous initiation of atrial fibrillation by ectopic beats originating from the pulmonary veins. *N Engl J Med* 1998; **339**: 659–66.

8 Tsai CF, Tai CT, Hsieh MH *et al*. Initiation of atrial fibrillation by ectopic beats originating from the superior vena cava: electrophysiological characteristics and results of radio-frequency ablation. *Circulation* 2000; **102**: 67–74.

9 Saksena S, Prakash A, Krol RB, Shankar A. Regional endocardial mapping of spontaneous and induced atrial fibrillation in patients with heart disease and refractory atrial fibrillation. *Am J Cardiol* 1999; **84**: 880–9.

10 Bennett MA, Pentecost BL. The pattern of onset and spontaneous cessation of atrial fibrillation in man. *Circulation* 1970; **41**: 981–8.

11 Chen SA, Tai CT, Yu WC *et al*. Right atrial focal atrial fibrillation: electrophysiologic characteristics and radiofrequency catheter ablation. *J Cardiovasc Electrophysiol* 1999; **10**: 328–35.

12 Oral H, Knight BP, Tada H *et al*. Pulmonary vein isolation for paroxysmal and persistent atrial fibrillation. *Circulation* 2002; **105**: 1077–81.

13 Chen SA, Hsieh MH, Tai CT *et al*. Initiation of atrial fibrillation by ectopic beats originating from the pulmonary veins: electrophysiological characteristics, pharmacological responses, and effects of radiofrequency ablation. *Circulation* 1999; **100**: 1879–86.

14 Chen YJ, Chen SA, Chen YC *et al*. Effects of rapid atrial pacing on the arrhythmogenic activity of single cardiomyocytes from pulmonary veins: implication in initiation of atrial fibrillation. *Circulation* 2001; **104**: 2849–54.

15 Hocini M, Ho SY, Kawara T *et al*. Electrical conduction in canine pulmonary veins. Electro-physiological and anatomic correlation. *Circulation* 2002; **105**: 2442–8.

16 Arora R, Verheule S, Scott L *et al*. Arrhythmogenic substrate of the pulmonary veins assessed by high resolution optical mapping. *Circulation* 2003; **107**: 1816–21.

17 Shah DC, Haissaguerre M, Jais P, Clementy J. High-resolution mapping of tachycardia originating from the superior vena cava: evidence of electrical heterogeneity, slow conduction and possible circus movement reentry. *J Cardiovasc Electrophysiol* 2002; **13**: 388–92.

18 Goya M, Ouyang F, Ernst S *et al*. Electroanatomic mapping and catheter ablation of break-throughs from the right atrium to the superior vena cava in patients with atrial fibrillation. *Circulation* 2002; **106**: 1317–20.

19 Doshi RN, Wu TJ, Yashima M *et al*. Relation between ligament of Marshall and adrenergic atrial tachyarrhythmia. *Circulation* 1999; **100**: 876–83.

20 Hwang C, Wu TJ, Doshi RN, Peter CT, Chen PS. Vein of Marshall cannulation for the analysis of electrical activity in patients with focal atrial fibrillation. *Circulation* 2000; **101**: 1503–5.

21 Kim DT, Lai AC, Hwang C *et al*. The ligament of Marshall: a structural analysis in human hearts with implications for atrial arrhythmias. *J Am Coll Cardiol* 2000; **36**: 1324–7.

22 Chen YJ, Chen SA, Chang MS, Lin CI. Arrhythmogenic activity of cardiac muscle in pulmonary veins of the dog: implication for the genesis of atrial fibrillation. *Cardiovasc Res* 2000; **48**: 265–73.

23 Chen YJ, Chen YC, Yeh HI, Lin CI, Chen SA. Electrophysiology and arrhythmogenic activity of single cardiomyocytes from canine superior vena cava. *Circulation* 2002; **105**: 2679–85.

24 Jais P, Hocini M, Macle L *et al.* Distinctive electrophysiological properties of pulmonary veins in patients with atrial fibrillation. *Circulation* 2002; **106**: 2479–85.

25 Nattel S. New ideas about atrial fibrillation 50 years on. *Nature* 2002; **415**: 219–26.

26 Wang J, Liu L, Feng J, Nattel S. Regional and functional factors determining induction and maintenance of atrial fibrillation in dogs. *Am J Physiol* 1996; **271**: H148–58.

27 Pappone C, Oreto G, Rosanio S *et al.* Atrial electroanatomic remodeling after circumferential radiofrequency pulmonary vein ablation: efficacy of an anatomic approach in a large cohort of patients with atrial fibrillation. *Circulation* 2001; **104**: 2539–44.

28 Tada H, Oral H, Ozaydin M *et al.* Response of pulmonary vein potentials to premature stimulation. *J Cardiovasc Electrophysiol* 2002; **13**: 33–7.

29 Knight BP, Oral H, Morady F. Paroxysmal fibrillation within an isolated pulmonary vein. *Circulation* 2002; **106**: 1426–7.

30 Tse HF, Pelosi F, Oral H *et al.* Effects of simultaneous atrioventricular pacing on atrial refractoriness and atrial fibrillation inducibility: role of atrial mechanoelectrical feedback. *J Cardiovasc Electrophysiol* 2001; **12**: 43–50.

31 Ravelli F, Allessie M. Effects of atrial dilatation on refractory period and vulnerability to atrial fibrillation in the isolated Langendorff-perfused rabbit heart. *Circulation* 1997; **96**: 1686–95.

32 Bosch RF, Nattel S. Cellular electrophysiology of atrial fibrillation. *Cardiovasc Res* 2002; **54**: 259–69.

33 Levine JH, Guarnieri T, Kadish AH, White RI, Calkins H, Kan JS. Changes in myocardial repolarization in patients undergoing balloon valvuloplasty for congenital pulmonary stenosis: evidence for contraction-excitation feedback in humans. *Circulation* 1988; **77**: 70–7.

34 Bode F, Sachs F, Franz MR. Tarantula peptide inhibits atrial fibrillation. *Nature* 2001; **409**: 35–6.

35 Fan K, Lee KL, Chow WH, Chau E, Lau CP. Internal cardioversion of chronic atrial fibrillation during percutaneous mitral commissurotomy: insight into reversal of chronic stretch-induced atrial remodeling. *Circulation* 2002; **105**: 2746–52.

36 Le Grand BL, Hatem S, Deroubaix E, Couetil JP, Coraboeuf E. Depressed transient outward and calcium currents in dilated human atria. *Cardiovasc Res* 1994; **28**: 548–56.

37 Behar S, Tanne D, Zion M *et al*, for the SPRINT study group. Incidence and prognostic significance of chronic atrial fibrillation among 5,839 consecutive patients with acute myocardial infarction. *Am J Cardiol* 1992; **70**: 816–18.

38 Rathore SS, Berger AK, Weinfurt KP *et al.* Acute myocardial infarction complicated by atrial fibrillation in the elderly. Prevalence and outcomes. *Circulation* 2000; **101**: 969–74.

39 Goldberg RJ, Yarzebski J, Lessard D, Wu J, Gore JM. Recent trends in the incidence rates of and death rates from atrial fibrillation complicating initial acute myocardial infarction: a community-wide perspective. *Am Heart J* 2002; **143**: 519–27.

40 Sakata K, Kurihara H, Iwamori K *et al.* Clinical and prognostic of atrial fibrillation in acute myocardial infarction. *Am J Cardiol* 1997; **80**: 1522–7.

41 Rechavia E, Strasberg B, Mager A *et al.* The incidence of atrial arrhythmias during inferior wall myocardial infarction with and without ventricular involvement. *Am Heart J* 1992; **124**: 387–91.

42 Nagahama Y, Suguira T, Takehana K *et al.* The role of infarction-associated pericarditis on the occurrence of atrial fibrillation. *Eur Heart J* 1998; **19**: 287–92.

43 Kamkin A, Kiseleva I, Wagner KD *et al.* Mechano-electrical feedback in right atrium after left ventricular infarction in rats. *J Mol Cell Cardiol* 2000; **32**: 465–77.

44 Sinno H, Derakhchan K, Libersan D *et al.* Atrial ischemia promotes atrial fibrillation in dogs. *Circulation* 2003; **107**: 1930–6.

45 Janse MJ, Wit AL. Electrophysiological mechanisms of ventricular arrhythmias resulting from myocardial ischemia and infarction. *Physiol Rev* 1989; **69**: 1049–169.

46 Braunwald E. Shattuck lecture – cardiovascular medicine at the turn of the millennium: triumphs, concerns, and opportunities. *N Engl J Med* 1997; **337**: 1360–9.

47 Ehrlich JR, Nattel S, Hohnloser SH. Atrial fibrillation and congestive heart failure: specific considerations at the intersection of two common and important cardiac disease sets. *J Cardiovasc Electrophysiol* 2002; **13**: 399–405.

48 Li D, Fareh S, Leung TK, Nattel S. Promotion of atrial fibrillation by heart failure in dogs – atrial remodeling of a different kind. *Circulation* 1999; **100**: 87–95.

49 Derakhchan K, Li D, Courtemanche M, Smith B, Brouillette J, Page PL, Nattel S. Method for simultaneous epicardial and endocardial mapping of in vivo canine heart: application to atrial conduction properties and arrhythmia mechanisms. *J Cardiovasc Electrophysiol* 2001; **12**: 548–55.

50 Li D, Melnyk P, Feng J *et al.* Effects of experimental heart failure on atrial cellular and ionic electrophysiology. *Circulation* 2000; **101**: 2631–8.

51 Coumel P. Clinical approach to paroxysmal atrial fibrillation. *Clin Cardiol* 1990; **13**: 209–12.

52 Schuessler RB, Grayson TM, Bromberg BI, Cox JL, Boineau JP. Cholinergically mediated tachyarrhythmias induced by a single extrastimulus in the isolated canine right atrium. *Circ Res* 1992; **71**: 1254–67.

53 Kneller J, Zou R, Vigmond EJ, Wang Z, Leon LJ, Nattel S. Cholinergic atrial fibrillation in a computer model of a two-dimensional sheet of canine atrial cells with realistic ionic properties. *Circ Res* 2002; **90**: E73–87.

54 Yamashita T, Murakawa Y, Hayami N *et al.* Relation between aging and circadian variation of paroxysmal atrial fibrillation. *Am J Cardiol* 1998; **82**: 1364–7.

55 Bettoni M, Zimmermann M. Autonomic tone variations before the onset of paroxysmal atrial fibrillation. *Circulation* 2002; **105**: 2753–9.

56 Bosch RF, Wang Z, Li GR, Nattel S. Electrophysiologic mechanisms by which hypothyroidism delays repolarization in guinea pig hearts. *Am J Physiol* 1999; **277**: H211–20.

57 Le Bouter S, Demolombe S, Chambellan A *et al.* Microarray analysis reveals complex remodeling of cardiac ion channel expression with altered thyroid status: relation to cellular and integrated electrophysiology. *Circ Res* 2003; **92**: 234–42.

58 Nattel S. The pathophysiology of atrial fibrillation. *Cardiac Electrophysiol Rev* 2001; **5**: 162–5.

59 Nattel S. Therapeutic implications of atrial fibrillation mechanisms: can mechanistic insights be used to improve AF management? *Cardiovasc Res* 2002; **54**: 347–60.

60 Wijffels MC, Kirchhof CJ, Dorland R, Allessie MA. Atrial fibrillation begets atrial fibrillation: a study in awake chronically instrumented goats. *Circulation* 1995; **92**: 1954–68.

61 Yue L, Feng J, Gaspo R, Li GR, Wang Z, Nattel S. Ionic remodeling underlying action potential changes in a canine model of atrial fibrillation. *Circ Res* 1997; **81**: 512–25.

62 Bosch RF, Zeng X, Grammer JB *et al.* Ionic mechanisms of electrical remodeling in human atrial fibrillation. *Cardiovasc Res* 1999; **44**: 121–31.

63 Goette A, Honeycutt C, Langberg JJ. Electrical remodeling in atrial fibrillation. Time course and mechanisms. *Circulation* 1996; **94**: 2968–74.

64 Sun H, Gaspo R, Leblanc N, Nattel S. Cellular mechanisms of atrial contractile dysfunction caused by sustained atrial tachycardia. *Circulation* 1998; **98**: 719–27.

65 Yue L, Melnyk P, Gaspo R, Wang Z, Nattel S. Molecular mechanisms underlying ionic remodeling in a dog model of atrial fibrillation. *Circ Res* 1999; **84**: 776–84.

66 Shinagawa K, Li D, Leung TK, Nattel S. Consequences of atrial tachycardia-induced remodeling depend on the preexisting atrial substrate. *Circulation* 2002; **105**: 251–7.

67 van der Velden HM, Ausma J, Rook MB *et al*. Gap junctional remodeling in relation to stabilization of atrial fibrillation in the goat. *Cardiovasc Res* 2000; **46**: 476–86.

68 Elvan A, Huang XD, Pressler ML, Zipes DP. Radiofrequency catheter ablation of the atria eliminates pacing-induced sustained atrial fibrillation and reduces connexin 43 in dogs. *Circulation* 1997; **96**: 1675–85.

69 Allessie M, Ausma J, Schotten U. Electrical, contractile and structural remodeling during atrial fibrillation. *Cardiovasc Res* 2002; **54**: 230–46.

70 Israel CW, Ehrlich JR, Gronefeld G *et al*. Prevalence, characteristics and clinical implications of regular atrial tachyarrhythmias in patients with atrial fibrillation: insights from a study using a new implantable device. *J Am Coll Cardiol* 2001; **38**: 355–63.

71 Oral H, Knight BP, Ozaydin M *et al*. Segmental ostial ablation to isolate the pulmonary veins during atrial fibrillation: feasibility and mechanistic insights. *Circulation* 2002; **106**: 1256–62.

72 Oral H, Knight BP, Tada H *et al*. Pulmonary vein isolation for paroxysmal and persistent atrial fibrillation. *Circulation* 2002; **105**: 1077–81.

73 Lee SH, Yu WC, Cheng JJ *et al*. Effect of verapamil on long-term tachycardia-induced atrial electrical remodeling. *Circulation* 2000; **101**: 200–6.

74 Fareh S, Benardeau A, Thibault B, Nattel S. The T-type Ca(2+) channel blocker mibefradil prevents the development of a substrate for atrial fibrillation by tachycardia-induced atrial remodeling in dogs. *Circulation* 1999; **100**: 2191–7.

75 Benardeau A, Fareh S, Nattel S. Effects of verapamil on atrial fibrillation and its electrophysiological determinants in dogs. *Cardiovasc Res* 2001; **50**: 85–96.

76 Kurita Y, Mitamura H, Shiroshita-Takeshita A *et al*. Daily oral verapamil before but not after rapid atrial excitation prevents electrical remodeling. *Cardiovasc Res* 2002; **54**: 447–55.

77 Nakashima H, Kumagai K, Urata H *et al*. Angiotensin II antagonist prevents electrical remodeling in atrial fibrillation. *Circulation* 2000; **101**: 2612–17.

78 Jayachandran JV, Zipes DP, Weksler J, Olgin JE. Role of the Na(+)/H(+) exchanger in short-term atrial electrophysiological remodeling. *Circulation* 2000; **101**: 1861–6.

79 Shinagawa K, Mitamura H, Ogawa S, Nattel S. Effects of inhibiting Na(+)/H(+)-exchange or angiotensin converting enzyme on atrial tachycardia-induced remodeling. *Cardiovasc Res* 2002; **54**: 438–46.

80 Yu WC, Lee SH, Tai CT *et al*. Reversal of atrial electrical remodeling following cardioversion of long-standing atrial fibrillation in man. *Cardiovasc Res* 1999; **42**: 470–6.

81 Nishino M, Hoshida S, Tanouchi J *et al*. Time to recover from atrial hormonal, mechanical, and electrical dysfunction after successful electrical cardioversion of persistent atrial fibrillation. *Am J Cardiol* 2000; **85**: 1451–4.

82 Everett TH, Li H, Mangrum JM *et al*. Electrical, morphological, and ultrastructural remodeling and reverse remodeling in a canine model of chronic atrial fibrillation. *Circulation* 2000; **102**: 1454–60.

83 Shinagawa K, Shiroshita-Takeshita A, Schram G, Nattel S. Effects of antiarrhythmic drugs on fibrillation in the remodeled atrium: insights into the mechanism of amiodarone's superior efficacy. *Circulation* 2003; **107**: 1440–6.

84 Zarse M, Stellbrink C, Athanatou E, Robert J, Schotten U, Hanrath P. Verapamil prevents stretch-induced shortening of atrial effective refractory period in langendorff-perfused rabbit heart. *J Cardiovasc Electrophysiol* 2001; **12**: 85–92.

85 Li D, Shinagawa K, Pang L *et al.* Effects of angiotensin-converting enzyme inhibition on the development of the atrial fibrillation substrate in dogs with ventricular tachypacing-induced congestive heart failure. *Circulation* 2001; **104**: 2608–14.

86 Shi Y, Li D, Tardif JC, Nattel S. Enalapril effects on atrial remodeling and atrial fibrillation in experimental congestive heart failure. *Cardiovasc Res* 2002; **54**: 456–61.

87 Shinagawa K, Shi YF, Tardif JC, Leung TK, Nattel S. Dynamic nature of atrial fibrillation substrate during development and reversal of heart failure in dogs. *Circulation* 2002; **105**: 2672–8.

88 Li D, Benardeau A, Nattel S. Contrasting efficacy of dofetilide in differing experimental models of atrial fibrillation. *Circulation* 2000; **102**: 104–12.

89 Pedersen OD, Bagger H, Keller N *et al.* Efficacy of dofetilide in the treatment of atrial fibrillation-flutter in patients with reduced left ventricular function: a Danish Investigations of Arrhythmia and Mortality on Dofetilide (DIAMOND) Substudy. *Circulation* 2001; **104**: 292–6.

90 Pedersen OD, Bagger H, Kober L, Torp-Pedersen C, on behalf of the TRACE study group. Trandopril reduces the incidence of atrial fibrillation after acute myocardial infarction in patients with left ventricular dysfunction. *Circulation* 1999; **100**: 376–80.

91 Cox JL, Ad N, Palazzo T *et al.* Current status of the Maze procedure for the treatment of atrial fibrillation. *Semin Thorac Cardiovasc Surg* 2000; **12**: 15–19.

92 Kottkamp H, Hindricks G, Autschbach R *et al.* Specific linear left atrial lesions in atrial fibrillation: intraoperative radiofrequency ablation using minimally invasive surgical techniques. *J Am Coll Cardiol* 2002; **40**: 475–80.

93 Cheung DW. Pulmonary vein as an ectopic focus in digitalis-induced arrhythmia. *Nature* 1981; **294**: 582–4.

94 Chen YJ, Chen SA, Chen YC *et al.* Electrophysiology of single cardiomyocytes isolated from rabbit pulmonary veins: implication in initiation of focal atrial fibrillation. *Basic Res Cardiol* 2002; **97**: 26–34.

95 Wang TM, Chiang CE, Sheu JR, Tsou CH, Chang HM, Luk HN. Homogeneous distribution of fast response action potentials in canine pulmonary vein sleeves: a contradictory report. *Int J Cardiol* 2003; **89**: 187–95.

CHAPTER 2

Neurological Basis of Atrial Fibrillation

Vladimir Shusterman, David Schwartzman

That an important, independent role exists for neural activity (healthy or pathological) in the development of atrial fibrillation (AF) in man has long been hypothesized. In this chapter we review the evidence to support this hypothesis and speculate about ways in which the brain–heart connection might be manipulated so as to reduce the AF burden.

Basic neuroatriology

The atria interface with sympathetic (adrenergic) and vagal nerve terminals, but their spatial distribution is not uniform [1]. Vagal terminals are predominantly found endocardially, whereas sympathetic terminals are found both endocardially and epicardially [2]. Vagal and sympathetic nerve stimulation each can shorten the atrial refractory period duration, but their effects are not territorially symmetrical [1, 2]. Vagal stimulation increases the heterogeneity of refractoriness, whereas sympathetic stimulation does not [3]. This is probably due to the inhomogeneity of vagal nerve distribution and nerve terminal acetylcholine concentration [4, 5]. In experimental preparations, the heterogeneity of refractoriness has been a key to the promotion of AF. Vagal and adrenergic terminals may also interact with one another. For example, acetylcholine released from vagal nerve endings diminishes the release of norepinephrine in adjacent sympathetic nerves [6]. Of course, interaction influencing nerve terminal activity also occurs at a distance, both peripherally and centrally [7]. Latency and duration of atrial electrophsyiological responses to vagal or adrenergic stimulation differ. Whereas the vagal response occurs within a few milliseconds, the adrenergic response is far slower [8]. In association with territorial heterogeneity, these differences may promote AF [9–11]. Prystowsky *et al.* demonstrated abbreviation of atrial refractoriness in patients during carotid baroreceptor stimulation (neck suction), which promotes vagotonia [12]. Shauerte *et al.* demonstrated that stimulation of cervical vagus nerve or the right pulmonary artery fat pad (a distribution center for atrial vagal neurons) produced regionally heterogeneous shortening of atrial refractoriness [13]. These effects were abolished with catheter ablation of the fat pad [14]. Interestingly, their abolition also diminished AF inducibility [14]. Pharmacological manipulation of atrial neural traffic has also been reported. For example, phenylephrine produces vagotonia and sympathetic withdrawal due to vasoconstriction, prolonging atrial refractoriness. This has been correlated with suppression of AF triggering by arrhythmogenic ectopy [15]. By contrast, proarrhythmic fertilization of the atrial substrate via enhanced heterogeneity in atrial conduction and refractoriness may occur after phenylephrine administration [16]. Isoproterenol may provoke atrial ectopy, suggesting that increased adrenergic force may enhance atrial automaticity [15]. Combined with diffuse abbreviation of conduction and refractoriness, this may explain the proarrhythmic effect of this drug in some patients. Inherent differences in atrial neural structure and function appear to influence atrial electrophysiology. For example, examining patients with supraventricular tachycardia, Chen *et al.* reported that baroreflex sensitivity was correlated with refractory period dispersion and propensity to AF [17, 18]. Observations such as these raise the question of whether there are neural phenotypes that favor the development of AF.

Evidence for neural influence on AF triggering and sustenance in man

As will be reviewed in detail below, sinus node activity has been the primary window to cardioneural interaction. Before proceeding, however, it is important to caution that it is not as yet clear that sinus node activity is adequate to portray the presence and magnitude of exchanges occurring between the nervous and cardiac systems. With respect to AF, it is possible that critical exchanges which affect triggering and/or sustenance occur which are not reflected by changes in sinus rate, possibly because of regional 'wiring' that does not involve the sinus node. It is also possible that specific changes in sinus rate do not consistently denote a given cardioneural milieu within or between individuals. In addition, it is not clear that quantification techniques applied to date adequately conceptualize or characterize what is actually occurring. Finally, and more practically, sinus node behavior is also influenced by non-neural elements, including intrinsic and humoral, and as such may be a transducer of variable (unpredictable) veracity. Nevertheless, many investigators have based mechanistic insights into the analysis of sinus node activity in the period preceding AF.

Coumel's seminal work classified AF into 'vagal' and 'adrenergic' subtypes [19, 20]. Patients plagued by the vagal subtype tend to describe onset at night and/or postprandially, as well as after exercise. These are times of vagal predominance, as defined by measures of heart rate variability (see below). Maneuvers that enhance vagal tone can sometimes provoke AF episodes, whereas exercise may be associated with their termination. Classically, vagal AF occurs in young (30- to 50-year-old) men without structural heart disease. By contrast, patients plagued by the adrenergic subtype of AF tend to describe onset during the daytime, particularly in the morning, and often during times of physical or mental stress. These are times of adrenergic predominance. Maneuvers that enhance sympathetic activity, can provoke events, whereas antiadrenergic measures such as beta blockade may suppress them. Methods utilizing sinus rate for assessment of neural activity take advantage of the fact that the vagal response time is shorter than the adrenergic response time. The two branches thus are readily separated in the frequency domain. Using the Fourier transform, a given period of electrocardiographic activity can be converted into a 'power spectrum', which presents rate variations as a spectrum of frequencies and magnitudes at which those frequencies occur (power). Experimental studies have shown that vagolysis blocks both low- (0.04–0.15 Hz) and high-frequency (0.15–0.4 Hz) range oscillation, whereas adrenergic blockade reduces the low-frequency oscillation only [21]. These observations led to the identification of a predominantly vagal high-frequency band and a 'mixed' adrenergic/vagal low-frequency band. Real-time tracking of changes in the power spectrum could provide a dynamic assessment of cardioneural interaction. Although human application is limited by confounding factors, including variable respiration frequency and physical activity, power spectral analysis has been widely used for the analysis of ANS activity in experimental and clinical studies and has led to interesting but often inconsistent results. For example, Vikman *et al.* analyzed sinus rate activity during 120 minutes preceding each of 92 AF episodes in 22 patients without a structural heart disease [22]. The number of atrial ectopic beats increased during 40 minutes before the event, whereas the approximate entropy (a measure of cardiac rhythm regularity [a time series containing repetitive patterns has a relatively small approximate entropy (ApEn), whereas random data yield higher values of ApEn]) [23] and α_1-scaling exponent (an estimate of the correlation properties of the cardiac rhythm) decreased before the onset. These measures applied to the pre-AF data were significantly lower than when applied to electrocardiographic data obtained from a matched group of healthy subjects. The authors concluded that decreases in complexity of sinus node activity precede the onset of AF in these patients. In a subsequent study, they also found that the high-frequency power (higher) and the low-frequency power and α_1-scaling exponent (lower) correlated with the duration of a given AF episode, possibly suggesting a role (in addition to fomenting AF triggering) for neural force in determining atrial substrate susceptibility to AF sustenance (see below). A decrease in the heart rate complexity, quantified by approximate entropy, and an increase in heart rate was also found in an hour before the onset of AF after coronary artery bypass graft surgery. However, changes in the high- and low-frequency heart rate variability power before the events were not uniform, suggesting involvement of mixed vagal and adrenergic mechanisms [22].

A circadian pattern of AF triggering is also well documented. For example, Yamashita *et al.* reported that AF triggering occurred more frequently after lunch and nocturnally [24]. Episodes beginning at night lasted significantly longer. Viskin *et al.* reported two peaks of AF onset, in the morning and in the evening, and concluded that the circadian rhythm of paroxysmal AF is similar to that for other cardiovascular diseases [25]. Gillis *et al.* observed two peaks of AF initiation, one in the early morning and one in the early evening hours [26]. In a large group of patients with implantable devices which provided full disclosure of AF frequency and time of onset, we examined the periodicity of AF onset and demonstrated that there was a distinct nocturnal preponderance (Fig. 2.1) [27]. Taken together, these data demonstrate that AF triggering

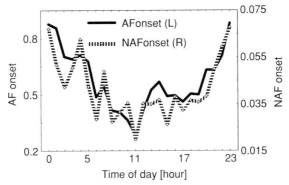

Fig. 2.1 Incidence of AF onset by time of day, as derived from information stored by implantable devices in a large cohort of patients. Raw (AF onset) and normalized (NAF onset) data are shown.

has a periodic pattern which can often but not always be correlated with a preponderance of vagal forces.

As has been detailed in other chapters in this book, ectopic atrial premature beats (APBs) are the dominant cause of AF triggering. A gradual increase in APB frequency and complexity is usually observed prior to AF onset, although emergence may occur suddenly. The cellular electrophysiological mechanism underlying the APB is probably afterdepolarization. It is possible that afterdepolarizations can be promoted by neural forces, either directly (e.g. neurochemical effect on myocyte transmembrane potential) or indirectly (e.g. myocyte effect caused by change in sinus rate magnitude or oscillation). In this regard, it is of interest that the dominant regions of origin of APBs which precipitate AF, left atrial myocardium within/contiguous to the pulmonary veins, are so richly interfaced with neural tissue. Invasive study in man has provided direct evidence of a link between neural forces and this region. During intracardiac electrophysiology study in man, Lu *et al.* contrasted AF episodes mediated by pulmonary vein APBs in which initiation was preceded by sinus cycle length oscillation, and contrasted these with other episodes which were initiated in association with a constant sinus cycle length [28]. The two types of the AF initiation were attributed to the distinct autonomic mechanisms. However, the short length of the analytical time window in this study (15 sinus cycles) was limiting. We examined longer-term (>10 minutes) changes in the sinus rate dynamics in a series of patients referred for catheter ablation of pulmonary vein APBs. Our data suggested a predominance of adrenergic forces preceding the onset of AF (Fig. 2.2). With regard to these insights, it should be emphasized that the artificial conditions and unique stresses inherent in invasive studies may limit their relevance to the native state.

In summary, the foregoing data strongly favor a key role for neural influence on AF. The preponderance of data suggest that triggering, mediated by promotion of atrial ectopy, is the principal means by which this occurs. However, there are also data to support the concept that neural forces can influence

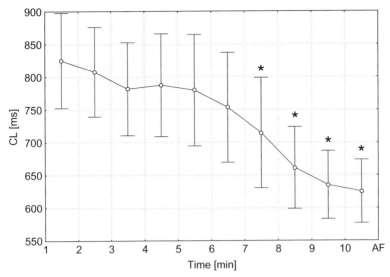

Fig. 2.2 Changes in the atrial cycle lengths preceding the onset of AF in the EP laboratory.
* $P < 0.05$ compared to min 1.

the atrial substrate so as to promote sustenance of AF. It is possible that neural involvement in AF is not pathological *per se*, rather a manifestation of physiological flux in autonomic tone during which susceptibility to fibrillation of a pathological atrial substrate varies. However, it is also possible that pathological neural forces are capable of playing a contributory role in AF promotion. If so, in individual patients these forces may be primary or secondary. For example, it is conceivable that in certain patients AF is a neurological disease, that is, mediated by intrinsically pathological neural signaling, mediated centrally or peripherally. Pathological signaling may be congenital or acquired. Contrarily, it is possible that pathological neural patterns are engendered by a disease acting upon the nervous system. Examples may include endocrinopathies, sleep apnea, and congestive heart failure.

Toward neurological therapy for AF

Although evidence supporting a neural role in promotion of AF seems solid, it is apparent from the foregoing discussion that there is heterogeneity as to how this occurs, both within and between individuals. Specifically, the data seem to support varied neural activity patterns preceding AF. Although it is possible that the neural heterogeneity is genuine, it is also possible that heterogeneity is introduced by the method used for analysis (e.g. the method misses the recurrent features). As noted above, it is also possible that the sinus node, the primary clinical window into cardiac neural activity, is an inconsistent or unreliable transducer. In thinking toward involving the nervous system in the quest for AF suppression, it is useful to separate the following conceptual roles.

Prediction

Toward this role we envision the development of techniques for real-time assessment of cardioneural activity patterns which would accurately portray the level of AF susceptibility. Advance warning of AF could then permit preemptive, intermittent introduction of pharmacological or non-pharmacological therapies (e.g. those which would not be feasible/tolerable if delivered tonically) to increase atrial resistance. Methods for the prediction of impending AF based on techniques summarized in the previous section would be unaccept-

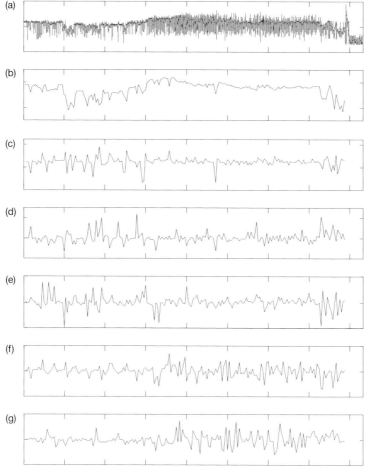

Fig. 2.3 Changes in the ventricular rhythm (a) and its most significant projections onto a set of individual fingerprint-basis vectors (b–g) 16 hours before the onset of paroxysmal AF. The variance of all projections was small during the first 4–5 hours, indicating stable rhythm and stable autonomic nervous system activity. However, during 8 hours before the onset of AF, the variance of the four projections increased and exceeded three standard deviations, indicating complex rhythm perturbations. AF started after 16 hours from the beginning of the recording.

Table 2.1 Dimensionality of the ventricular rhythm
disturbances as a predictor of the onset of AF

Dm	SE	SP	PA
≥4	80	93	92
≥3	87	67	72
≥2	1	40	63

SE = sensitivity; SP = specificity; PA = predictive accuracy.

able because of issues including diagnostic limitations and implementation
drawbacks:
• there is no accounting for individual features of cardiac rhythm, including
the pattern, range and variation
• the approach is applied blindly with respect to period, without estimation
of the temporal risk of AF
• there is no attempt to integrate multiple potentially relevant indicators (e.g.
number of APBs, heart rate, heart rate variability, power spectrum)
• the techniques use short windows to determine cardiac rhythm. Long-term
changes, which are usually more pronounced and complex than the short-
term variations, are ignored [29].

We hypothesized that accurate, real-time AF forecasting could be achieved
using an individualized method, in which specific variations from each patient's
own baseline cardioneural fingerprint correlates with their AF susceptibility. In
this method (tailored multifactorial cardioneural analysis [TMA]), the analytical
system learns the entire spectrum of the cardioneural activity for the individual,
including the heart rate, its oscillations, number and coupling of PACs, etc.,
and tracks any excursions from the characteristic pattern that might indicate
physiological instabilities. The method provides the tools for quantifying these
excursions according to their magnitude and the degree of deviation from the
characteristic pattern. We had previously used TMA in the analysis of cardioneural activity preceding the onset of ventricular tachyarrhythmias [30]. We
were able to identify subtle but highly specific changes in cardiac rhythm that
predict the onset of ventricular tachyarrhythmias. The technique proved more
accurate than the traditional indices described above. We have recently begun
to use TMA for AF forecasting. Retrospective analysis of ambulatory electrocardiographic recordings demonstrated excellent accuracy in portraying periods
of high AF risk (Fig. 2.3, Table 2.1) [31]. We found that the disturbances from
baseline cardioneural activity as characterized by the TMA technique gradually
increased several hours before the event (Fig. 2.4). Excluding the presence and
frequency of APBs from the input data reduced but did not eliminate the ability
of TMA to accurately forecast AF. As described above, APBs are a necessary component of AF triggering. Our forecasting experience suggests that APBs are
necessary but not sufficient to achieve AF onset. We thus speculate that initiation
of AF requires neural forces beyond those which are required to elicit APBs.

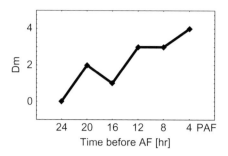

Fig. 2.4 Changes in the dimensionality (Dm) of the disturbances of ventricular rhythm before the onset of AF ($n = 15$).

Prevention

Toward this role we envision the development of techniques for active manipulation of neural forces acting on the heart. In that we believe cardioneural activity to be centrally coordinated, it is intriguing to speculate that brain-level therapies would be effective in AF prevention. In fact, we and others have demonstrated that cardioneural interaction can be altered by direct brain stimulation [32]. Modulation of brain activity by direct stimulation using implanted devices has been utilized for certain neurological disorders [33]. However, for multiple reasons the clinical application of such a technique for AF will probably never become reality. Conceptualization of therapies targeting peripheral nerve elements for this purpose is much more reasonable. One region which might be targeted could be the cervical spine, where surgical access to nerve trunks carrying cardiac vagal or sympathetic fibers projecting from the central nervous system is feasible. Chronic, intermittent stimulation of cervical nerve trunks using implanted devices has been used in the treatment of certain seizure disorders [34]. In our opinion, the most promising region for neurological AF intervention is in the region contiguous to the atria. As mentioned above, certain neurons traveling to the atria pass through areas contiguous to the atria which are anatomically identifiable (fat pads) and consistently located. It is reasonable to hypothesize that these areas could be targeted with minimally invasive techniques. For example, as detailed in Chapter 13, it is likely that pharmacological agents delivered transpericardially would have excellent access to periatrial neural elements. It is not unreasonable to speculate that among these agents might be neurotropic viral vectors capable of transfection with genes which would alter neural effects on the atrium. Similarly, it is possible that direct electrical stimulation, intermittent or tonic, could be applied to these areas. The concept of an implantable device which would combine automatic and/or patient-activated 'neural pacing' with real-time AF forecasting is particularly exciting. Finally, ablation of these areas is possible. Studies in animal models have shown that epicardium and endocardium-based techniques for ablation of periatrial neural elements using radiofrequency energy is feasible, and may have an antiarrhythmic effect [13]. In man, nascent information suggests that targeted surgical ablation can reduce the incidence of postoperative AF [35]. More recently, it has been suggested that successful outcome in patients undergoing radiofrequency catheter ablation of AF (see Chapter 7) can be correlated with vagal denervation [36]. This raises the interesting possibility that the therapeutic effect of posterior left atrial catheter ablation may be less dependent on the burden than on the (perineural) location of ablation lesions. Prospective clinical studies are under way to further explore this concept.

References

1 Tai CT, Chiou CW, Chen SA. Interaction between the autonomic nervous system and atrial tachyarrhythmias. *J Cardiovasc Electrophysiol* 2002; **13**: 83–7.
2 Marron K, Wharton J, Sheppard MN *et al*. Distribution, morphology, and neurochemistry of endocardial and epicardial nerve terminal arborations in the human heart. *Circulation* 1995; **92**: 2343–51.
3 Liu L, Nattel S. Differing sympathetic and vagal effects on atrial fibrillation in dogs: role of refractoriness heterogeneity. *Am J Physiol* 1997; **273**: H805–H816.
4 Olgin JE, Sih HJ, Hanish S *et al*. Heterogeneous atrial denervation creates substrate for sustained atrial fibrillation. *Circulation* 1998; **98**: 2608–14.
5 Jayachandran JV, Sih HJ, Winkle W *et al*. Atrial fibrillation produced by prolonged rapid atrial pacing is associated with heterogeneous changes in atrial sympathetic innervation. *Circulation* 2000; **101**: 1188–91.
6 Levy MN. Autonomic interactions in cardiac control. In: Coumel P, Garfein OB, eds. *Electrocardiography: Past and Future*, 1990: 209–21.
7 Shusterman V, Jannetta PJ, Aysin B *et al*. Direct mechanical stimulation of brainstem modulates cardiac rhythm and repolarization in humans. *J Electrocardiol* 2002; **35**: 247–56.
8 Coumel P. Neural aspects of paroxysmal atrial fibrillation. In: Falk RH, Podrid PJ, eds. *Atrial Fibrillation: Mechanisms and Management*. New York: Raven Press, 1992: 109–25.
9 Ninomyia I. Direct evidence of nonuniform distribution of vagal effects on dog atria. *Circ Res* 1966; **19**: 576–83.
10 Armour JA, Murphy DA, Yuan BX, Macdonald S, Hopkins DA. Gross and microscopic anatomy of the human intrinsic cardiac nervous system. *Anat Rec* 1997; **247**: 289–98.
11 Randall WC. Sympathetic modulation of normal cardiac rhythm. In: Rosen MR, Janse MJ, Wit AL, eds. *Cardiac Electrophysiology*. Mount Kisco, NY: Futura, 1990: 889–901.
12 Prystowsky EN, Naccarelli GV, Jackman WN *et al*. Enhanced parasympathetic tone shortens atrial refractoriness in man. *Am J Cardiol* 1983; **51**: 96–100.
13 Schauerte P, Scherlag BJ, Patterson E *et al*. Focal atrial fibrillation: experimental evidence for a pathophysiologic role of the autonomic nervous system. *J Cardiovasc Electrophysiol* 2001; **12**: 592–9.
14 Schauerte P, Scherlag BJ, Pitha J *et al*. Catheter ablation of cardiac autonomic nerves for prevention of vagal atrial fibrillation. *Circulation* 2000; **102**: 2774–80.
15 Tai CT, Chiou CW, Wen ZC *et al*. Effects of phenylephrine on focal atrial fibrillation originating in the pulmonary veins and superior vena cava. *J Am Coll Cardiol* 2000; **36**: 788–93.
16 Leitch JW, Basta M, Fletcher PJ. Effect of phenylephrine infusion on atrial electrophysiologic properties. *Heart* 1997; **78**: 166–70.
17 Chen YJ, Chen SA, Tai CT *et al*. Role of atrial electrophysiology and autonomic nervous system in patients with supraventricular tachycardia and paroxysmal atrial fibrillation. *J Am Coll Cardiol* 1998; **32**: 732–8.

18 Chen YJ, Tai CT, Chiou CW *et al*. Inducibility of atrial fibrillation during atrioventricular pacing with varying intervals: Role of atrial electrophysiology and the autonomic nervous system. *J Cardiovasc Electrophysiol* 1999; **10**: 1578–85.

19 Coumel P. Neural aspects of paroxysmal atrial fibrillation. In: Falk RH, Podrid PJ, eds. *Atrial Fibrillation: Mechanisms and Management*. New York: Raven Press, 1992: 109–25.

20 Coumel P. Autonomic arrhythmogenic factors in paroxysmal atrial fibrillation. In: Olsson SB, Alessie MA, eds. *Atrial Fibrillation: Mechanisms and Therapeutic Strategies*. Armonk, NY: Futura Publishing, 1994: 171–85.

21 Huang JL, Wen ZC, Lee WL, Chang MS, Chen SA. Changes of autonomic tone before the onset of paroxysmal atrial fibrillation. *Int J Cardiol* 1998; **66**: 275–83.

22 Vikman S, Makikallio TH, Yli-Mayry S *et al*. Altered complexity and correlation properties of R-R interval dynamics before the spontaneous onset of paroxysmal atrial fibrillation. *Circulation* 1999; **100**: 2079–84.

23 Pincus SM. Approximate entropy as a measure of system complexity. *Proc Natl Acad Sci U S A* 1991; **88**: 2297–301.

24 Yamashita T. Murakawa Y, Sezaki K *et al*. Circadian variation of paroxysmal atrial fibrillation. *Circulation* 1997; **96**: 1537–41.

25 Viskin S, Golovner M, Malov N *et al*. Circadian variation of symptomatic paroxysmal atrial fibrillation. Data from almost 10,000 episodes. *Eur Heart J* 1999; **20**: 1429–34.

26 Gillis AM, Connolly SJ, Dubuc M *et al*. and PA3 Investigators. Circadian variation of paroxysmal atrial fibrillation. Atrial Pacing Peri-ablation for Prevention of Atrial Fibrillation Trial. *Am J Cardiol* 2001; **87**: 794–8.

27 Shusterman V, Warman E, Usiene I, Schaaf K, Schwartzman D. Patterns of initiation of paroxysmal atrial fibrillation [abstract]. *Circulation* 2002; **106**: 458.

28 Lu TM, Tai CT, Hsieh MH *et al*. Electrophysiologic characteristics in initiation of paroxysmal atrial fibrillation from a focal area. *J Am Coll Cardiol* 2001; **37**: 1658–64.

29 Shusterman V, Aysin B, Gottipaty V *et al*. for the ESVEM Investigators. Autonomic nervous system activity and the spontaneous initiation of ventricular tachycardia *J Am Coll Cardiol* 1998; **32**: 1891–9.

30 Shusterman V, Aysin B, Chaparro L *et al*. for the ESVEM Investigators. On-line prediction of ventricular tachyarrhythmias using short-term rr-interval perturbations: comparative analysis of different signal processing techniques. *PACE* 1999; **22**: 837.

31 Shusterman V, Aysin B, Weiss R *et al*. Changes in the pattern of cardiac cycle dynamics predict initiation of paroxysmal atrial fibrillation. *PACE* 2000; **23**: 668.

32 Shusterman V, Jannetta PJ, Aysin B *et al*. Direct mechanical stimulation of brainstem modulates cardiac rhythm and repolarization in humans. *J Electrocardiol* 2002; **35**: 247–56.

33 Goodman JH. Brain stimulation as therapy for epilepsy. *Adv Exp Med Biol* 2004; **548**: 239–47.

34 Wheless JW. Nonpharmacologic treatment of the catastrophic epilepsies of childhood. *Epilepsia* 2004; **45** (Suppl 5): 17–22.

35 Melo J, Voight P, Sonmez B *et al*. Ventral cardiac denervation reduces the incidence of atrial fibrillation after coronary artery bypass grafting. *J Thorac Cardiovasc Surg* 2004; **127**: 511–16.

36 Pappone C, Santinelli V, Manguso F *et al*. Pulmonary vein denervation enhances long-term benefit after circumferential ablation for paroxysmal atrial fibrillation. *Circulation* 2004; **109**: 327–34.

CHAPTER 3

Mechanical Basis of Atrial Fibrillation

Douglas A. Hettrick, David Schwartzman, Hung-Fat Tse, Paul S. Pagel

Overall cardiovascular performance is determined by the complex mechanical interaction of the preload or venous system and the afterload or arterial system, as well as the systolic and diastolic mechanical properties of the ventricles. These four distinct mechanical systems interact via the circulating blood volume. The atria are part of the preload system since they assist in ventricular filling and interact mechanically with the filling ventricles. The atria play three major mechanical roles: conduit, reservoir, and booster pump (contractility) [1]. Atrial conduit function encompasses the antegrade venous transport of blood from the pulmonary veins, or vena cava, through the atria and directly into the left and right ventricles, respectively, during the rapid filling and diastasis phases of ventricular diastole. Reservoir function encompasses the capacitance of the atria, including the appendages, to store returning venous blood volume while the mitral and tricuspid valves are closed. Atrial reservoir function makes a large volume of blood available to the ventricles at a low energy cost in order to maximize ventricular filling immediately after mitral or tricuspid valve opening. Booster pump function encompasses the active contraction of the atria, or atrial systole, to augment late ventricular filling. Atrial–ventricular coupling describes the relationship between the dynamic mechanical characteristics of the atria (e.g. elastance and viscosity) and those of the ventricles during filling. The physical dimensions of the mitral and tricuspid valves and the diastolic mechanical properties of the ventricles (e.g. compliance and viscoelasticity), determine the atrial afterload (e.g. ventricular input impedance). Thus, augmented atrial function alone may not enhance ventricular filling unless it is appropriately matched to ventricular input impedance.

Given that the left atrium (LA) appears to be the mechanistic seat of atrial fibrillation (AF), in this chapter we will focus on its mechanical function. We believe that abnormalities in mechanical function breed histopathologic changes which underlie the AF substrate. That AF is in essence a mechanical disease is supported by both animal models [2] and by epidemiologic features which link it to reduced vascular and left ventricular compliance [3, 4].

Quantification of left atrial mechanical function

Atrial function may be described by its relative contractile contribution to ventricular filling and cardiac output [5, 6]. Non-invasive assessment of LA function was initially described using transmitral or pulmonary venous (PV) blood flow velocity patterns, two-dimensional (2D) LA echocardiography, angiography or radionuclide imaging. More recently, evaluation of LA function has been performed using magnetic resonance imaging and electron beam computed tomography. These non-invasive techniques provide important clinical information about LA function beyond simple hemodynamic assessment. Direct invasive assessment of LA function using three-dimensional orthogonal sonomicrometry and high-fidelity measurement of LA pressure may only be conducted in the laboratory [7, 8]. These experimental determinations of continuous LA pressure and volume allow quantification of LA function in the pressure–volume plane using techniques adapted from left ventricle (LV) function analysis. Novel techniques for determining atrial dimensions, such as catheter contact mapping and chamber conductance, have the potential to provide additional clinical information about atrial function in patients.

The temporal LA pressure waveform consists of two major and one minor deflections during normal sinus rhythm (Fig. 3.1). LA contraction occurs after atrial depolarization and produces the 'a' wave at the end of LV diastole. Subsequent LV contraction causes a small retrograde pressure wave associated with mitral valve closure that results in a brief rise in LA pressure known as the 'c' wave. During the remainder of LV isovolumic contraction, ejection and isovolumic relaxation, blood flow from the PV fills the passive LA and gradually increases LA pressure. This volume increase results in the LA 'v' wave just before the mitral valve opens and early LV filling begins. The LA volume waveform is also polyphasic. When atrial tissue is relaxed, atrial volume lags pressure, but has analogous morphometry, also exhibiting a 'v' wave. That is, increased atrial pressure is associated with increased atrial volume. In contrast, atrial pressure increases in association with decreased atrial volume during atrial contraction. A 'c' wave associated with mitral valve closure may also be visible in the atrial pressure waveform (Fig. 3.1).

Atrial myocardium demonstrates time-varying viscoelastic mechanical properties. Myocardial viscosity determines energy loss due to friction and is manifest in myocardial tissue by mechanical phenomena such as creep, stretch relaxation and hysteresis. The amount of energy lost to friction by the atrial myocardium during the cardiac cycle depends on the viscosity of the myocardium itself, the viscosity of the blood, and the rate of atrial filling. That is, more energy loss occurs at higher rates of atrial filling and ejection. The term elastance, or stiffness, describes the change in atrial pressure associated with a given change in volume and is the mathematical inverse of compliance. Elastance changes during the cardiac mechanical cycle; it is higher during systole than during atrial relaxation, similar to the ventricular myocardium.

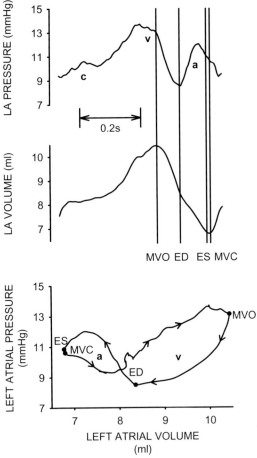

Fig. 3.1 Steady-state left atrial (LA) pressure–volume diagram for a single cardiac cycle. The 'a' portion of the diagram (left loop) incorporates active LA contraction and temporally proceeds in a counterclockwise fashion. The 'v' portion of the diagram (right loop) represents passive LA reservoir function and proceeds in a clockwise manner over time. Left atrial end-diastole and end-systole (ED and ES, respectively) and mitral valve closure and opening (MVC and MVO, respectively) are also depicted on the LA pressure–volume diagram. Left ventricular isovolumic contraction, ejection, and the majority of isovolumic relaxation occur during the time between MVC and MVO illustrated on the LA pressure–volume diagram. Arrows indicate the direction of movement around the diagram over time. 'c' indicates the pressure associated with mitral valve closure.

The LA pressure–volume relationship typically consists of a dual-loop morphology arranged in a figure-of-eight pattern because of the biphasic deflection morphology of the LA pressure and volume waveforms (Fig. 3.2). The LA pressure–volume diagram describes both the active (a) and passive (v) components of LA function. The active component of the diagram (a loop) begins at LA end-diastole (Fig. 3.1) and temporally progresses in a counterclockwise

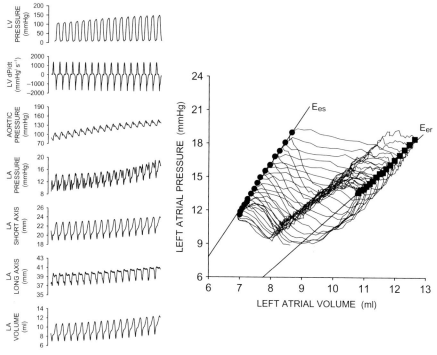

Fig. 3.2 Continuous left ventricular (LV) pressure, LV dP/dt, aortic pressure, left atrial (LA) pressure, LA short- and long-axis dimensions, and LA volume wave forms (left) and corresponding LA pressure–volume diagrams (right) resulting from intravenous administration of phenylephrine (200 μg). The LA maximum elastance (solid dots) and end-reservoir pressure and volume (solid squares) for each pressure–volume diagram are used to obtain the slopes (E_{es} and E_{er}) and extrapolated volume intercepts of the LA end-systolic and end-reservoir pressure–volume relations to quantify myocardial contractility and dynamic chamber stiffness, respectively.

manner as blood is ejected from the LA during atrial systole. Under normal conditions, a small volume of blood is ejected retrogradely into the pulmonary veins during atrial systole. This retrograde PV flow is substantially reduced by the peristaltic action of atrial contraction and the pseudo-valve-like anatomy of the PV–LA junction [9], but is not represented on the LA pressure–volume diagram. Atrial regurgitant blood flow into the PV increases during the LA hypertension that may accompany mitral stenosis or insufficiency, myocardial ischemia, or cardiomyopathy (see below). Retrograde pulmonary venous flow associated with atrial contraction is also an important marker of LV diastolic dysfunction that is assessed clinically using Doppler echocardiography. Atrial contraction ends at LA end-systole (Fig. 3.1) and LA filling then occurs during LV systole. Thus, LA stroke volume and emptying fraction may be calculated directly from the LA pressure–volume diagram. The area of the 'a' loop represents active LA stroke work performed by the atrium during atrial systole. As previously mentioned, this work may contribute to ventricular filling under conditions of optimized atrial–ventricular mechanical coupling. However, atrial stroke work may also result in enhanced retrograde pulmonary venous flow, particularly if atrial contraction is poorly timed or if the LV is very stiff. The passive component of the LA pressure–volume diagram, or 'v' loop, proceeds temporally in a clockwise direction. Thus, changes in LA pressure and volume that occur during this phase of the cardiac cycle result from external forces acting upon the viscoelastic atrial myocardium. The right ventricle presumably generates these forces by pumping blood into the pulmonary circulation. The area of the 'v' loop represents energy lost to viscosity and is also proportional to atrial reservoir function at constant atrial filling rate [8]. The slope of the line between minimal LA pressure of the 'a' loop and maximal pressure in the 'v' loop represents the passive filling curve of the atrium and may be used to assess steady-state LA compliance. The difference between minimal and maximal volume obtained from the 'a' and 'v' loops is LA reservoir volume [1].

Acute alterations in LA loading conditions produced by volume administration, mechanical occlusion of the vena cava or aorta, or pharmacological interventions, including bolus administration of phenylephrine, may be used to generate a series of differentially loaded LA pressure–volume diagrams for the assessment of LA contractility using the LA end-systolic pressure–volume relation (Fig. 3.2) [10]. Alterations in LA contractile state may be quantified with the slope (end-systolic elastance; Ees) of this LA end-systolic pressure–volume relationship, analogous to the well-established techniques commonly applied to the ventricle. The reservoir, conduit, and contractile properties of the LA are affected by LA relaxation [1, 11], compliance [12] and myocardial contractility [13, 14]. The LA acts as a reservoir for PV flow during LA relaxation, LV systole and the majority of LV relaxation (represented by the lower portion of the 'a' loop and the upper portion of the 'v' loop). Passive emptying of the LA occurs immediately after the mitral valve opens. The LA–LV pressure gradient determines the extent of early LV filling and is dependent on LA pressure, the degree of LV relaxation, and LV compliance. Delayed LV relaxation or increased LV stiffness reduce the LA–LV pressure gradient and hence, attenuate rapid LV filling. The LA then functions as a conduit to additional PV blood flow during LV diastasis (the final part of the 'v' loop and the initial part of the 'a' loop). The compliance of the passive atrial myocardium is a major determinant of LA filling and LV performance [15]. Reservoir function is determined by LA relaxation [1], LA chamber stiffness, descent of the cardiac base during LV systole, and the right ventricle systolic pressure pulse transmitted through the pulmonary venous circulation [11]. These factors combine to produce a biphasic PV blood flow pattern during LV systole. This process is most often observed with the S wave of PV blood flow velocity, commonly determined with Doppler echocardiography. A direct relation between LA compliance and LA reservoir function has been demonstrated in dogs and humans. Delayed LA relaxation or reduced LA compliance is associated

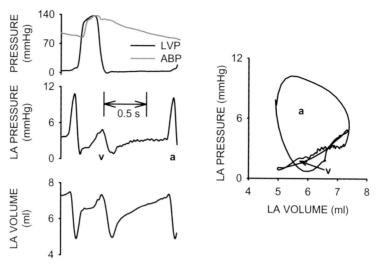

Fig. 3.3 Left ventricular and arterial pressures (top left), left atrial (LA) pressure (middle left), LA volume (bottom left), and the corresponding LA pressure–volume diagram (right) from a conscious dog with bradycardia and sinus arrhythmia. Prolonged diastasis allows the LA to completely refill before contraction. Note the large relative area of the active work ('a' loop) compared with the passive work ('v' loop).

with attenuated early reservoir function and a blunted S wave. Cardiac output and early LA reservoir function are related [16, 17] because LA filling during the early reservoir phase is a determinant of the extent of early LV filling. The rate and extent of early reservoir filling are substantially reduced by regional myocardial ischemia because LV systolic base descent is adversely affected [13, 14].

The morphology of the steady-state LA pressure–volume diagram may vary to some degree with heart rate or timing (Fig. 3.3). A prolonged cardiac cycle associated with bradycardia and sinus arrhythmia lengthens LV diastasis, resulting in extensive refilling of the LA after the mitral valve opens before the onset of atrial contraction. This refilling of the atria during prolonged diastasis produces an overlap of the 'a' and 'v' loops for a single cardiac cycle. In addition, mitral valve closure may occasionally be associated with a distinct 'c' loop, especially at short atrioventricular (AV) coupling intervals (Fig. 3.4). Mitral valve closure is manifest as a depression in the 'a' loop at different AV coupling intervals. Descent of the ventricular base may also exert an external pulling force on the atria, changing the temporal direction of the 'v' loop from a clockwise to a counterclockwise orientation. This may result in the appearance of an additional 'transition loop' during diastasis after completion of LV relaxation. Atrial contractile failure results in the absence of the 'a' loop despite increases in atrial pressure. Under these circumstances, atrial contraction is not associated with decreased volume (Fig. 3.5).

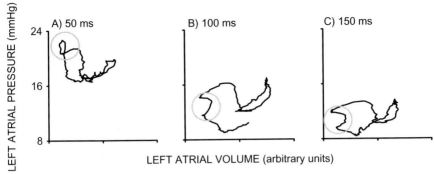

Fig. 3.4 Variations in atrial pressure–volume loop morphology. Effects of mitral valve timing are shown. These loops were acquired using the conductance catheter technique to determine relative chamber volume (arbitrary units) in one patient during dual-chamber pacing at various pressure–volume delays (A, 50 ms; B, 100 ms; C, 150 ms). The timing of mitral valve closure relative to atrial contraction is manifest by a depression in the left edge of the loop or by a distinct 'c' loop in part A (gray circles). The appearance of this 'c' loop may indicate reduced atrial–ventricular mechanical coupling.

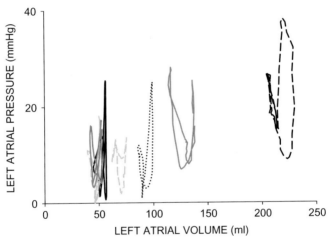

Fig. 3.5 Pseudo-steady-state left atrial pressure–volume loops obtained during contact mapping electrophysiological laboratory procedures from seven patients during normal sinus rhythm. Pressure–volume diagrams span a range of pressures and volumes, but nevertheless correspond to atrial function. In this figure, patients with lower pressure and volume may have significantly greater contractile atrial function compared with patients with higher pressure atria. The patient on the far right appears to have lost atrial pump function due to chronic atrial dilation and overload.

Clinical measurement of left atrial mechanical function

LA myocardial contractility has been quantified *in vivo* using LA pressure–volume analysis [10, 13]. Instantaneous LA pressure–volume relations based on a time-varying elastance model are relatively independent of loading conditions and are sensitive to alterations in the intrinsic inotropic state [10]. Such end-systolic pressure–volume relations have been used extensively in laboratory and clinical investigations to describe LV and LA contractility [13]. Ees derived from a series of end-systolic pressure–volume diagrams is most often used to quantify LA contractility [13]. The linearity of the LA end-systolic pressure–volume relation is clear from the high correlation coefficients generated using regression analysis (Fig. 3.2). LA Ees is highly reproducible, sensitive to calcium and volatile anesthetic-induced increases and decreases in LA contractility, respectively, and relatively simple to derive under controlled experimental conditions [13]. LA Ees has also been determined in humans using 2D echocardiography [12]. Decreased Ees has been observed in patients with congestive heart failure. Recently, conductance catheter technique for chamber volume measurement has been applied in the right atrium [18, 19] and left atrium (Fig. 3.4) to measure relative changes in atrial pressure–volume relationships. Electrophysiology laboratory contact mapping systems may also be useful in generating pseudo-steady-state LA pressure–volume diagrams (Fig. 3.5). Furthermore, new intra-chamber imaging modalities, such as intravenous ultrasound and tissue Doppler techniques, may provide additional measures of clinical atrial function.

LA afterload is determined by mitral valve resistance and LV compliance [20]. The mitral valve does not contribute substantially to afterload under normal circumstances. However, mitral valve resistance becomes the major factor in determining LA afterload during mitral stenosis. LA afterload progressively increases as LV compliance decreases. The relative contribution of the LA systole to LV end-diastolic volume depends on the timing of LA contraction, PV blood return during diastasis, autonomic nervous system activity, and LV diastolic pressure, compliance and functional reserve. Alterations in LA reservoir volume and 'v' loop areas are the strongest indicators of the LA contractile contribution to LV filling in normal hearts and those from patients with essential hypertension [1, 16]. Despite these data, the relative contribution of LA systole to LV filling remains difficult to quantify and has as yet undefined prognostic significance in patients with abnormal LV performance [16, 21]. The absence of easily measured indices of LA function has made resolution of this controversy difficult. LV adaptation to LA dysfunction has also not been extensively studied.

Mechanical coupling of atrium to ventricle

The ratio of LA Ees to effective LV elastance (Elv) describes the coupling between the LA and LV. This ratio is approximately equal to 1 in the normal heart [12], indicating that LA systolic energy transfer to the LV is appropriately matched. However, LA–LV coupling may be impaired in heart failure because compensatory increases in LA contractility do not overcome reductions in LV compliance. Such an increase in LA contractile function is known to occur in patients with ischemic or hypertensive heart disease [16, 22] that preserves LA–LV coupling early in the natural history of these diseases. Therapy directed at improving LV diastolic function (e.g. nitrates in acute regional myocardial ischemia or afterload reduction in pressure-overload hypertrophy) may improve LA–LV coupling. Again, lack of clinically accessible indices of LA contractility and LV compliance has complicated the evaluation of LA–LV coupling in patients with heart disease. Approaches based on a time-varying elastance model will be useful to describe LA contractile function and estimate Elv, which may be used in the cardiac catheterization laboratory.

Under normal conditions, atrial systole typically contributes 15–20% of LV stroke volume [6]. However, LA contractile function may contribute a greater percentage to ventricular filling and stroke volume in patients with heart failure. LA contractile function is enhanced early in the natural history of LV diastolic dysfunction. LV filling is preserved by augmented LA contractility in patients with impaired LV diastolic function, but chronic atrial overload may eventually lead to decreased atrial function (Fig. 3.6). Accordingly, patients with LV diastolic dysfunction may acutely develop heart failure when LA contractile function becomes exhausted or is eliminated entirely during tachyarrhythmias [5, 14, 23, 24]. Thus, restoration of LA function in these patients improves LV filling and performance and reduces the clinical signs and symptoms of heart failure [25]. Increases in LV diastolic pressure occurring during LV ischemia, infarction or overload may produce LA dilation or remodeling that subsequently reduces LA contractility, decreases LA compliance, and increases the likelihood of arrhythmias.

LA adaptation to LV diastolic dysfunction is incompletely understood. Increases in LA compliance initially occur as LA volume expands during LV diastolic dysfunction as a result of pacing-induced cardiomyopathy; however, LA Ees and emptying fraction are maintained [25, 26]. These data suggest that LA systolic function is preserved despite moderate dilation of the chamber during evolving heart failure. LA contractile function is eventually reduced as LV function worsens and LA afterload increases [27] (Fig. 3.7). LA stroke work requires greater energy expenditure because increased resistance to active emptying results from reduced LV compliance. Subsequently, LA contractile function becomes severely depressed and marked declines in the active LA contribution to LV stroke volume occur. Compensatory upregulation of the β-myosin isoform in atrial myocardium is associated with increased LA mechanical work in humans [28], but progressive LV diastolic dysfunction eventually contributes to LA failure. LA remodeling may also occur in response to decreases in LV compliance and contribute to exaggerated pressure responses to small increases in volume. Such remodeling of the LA restricts PV blood flow during the reservoir phase, leads to pulmonary venous congestion, and may produce clinical dyspnea. Continued research will be required to further our understanding of factors that affect atrial–ventricular mechanical coupling in the presence of ventricular dysfunction.

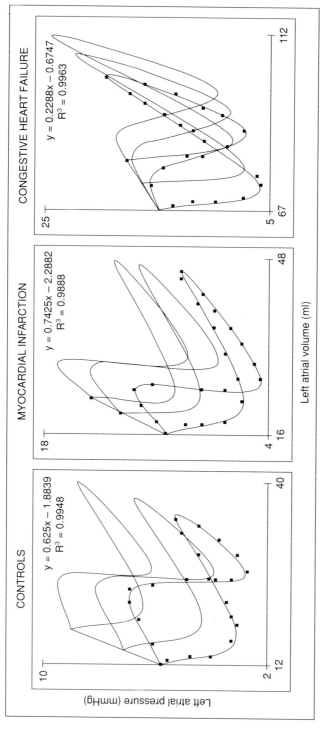

Fig. 3.6 Differentially loaded left atrial (LA) pressure–volume diagrams and LA end-systolic pressure–volume relations obtained during saline infusion in typical patients with normal cardiac function (left panel; controls) and those with left ventricular (LV) myocardial infarction (middle panel) and congestive heart failure (right panel). A compensatory increase in LA contractility (slope of the LA end-systolic pressure–volume relation) is observed in patients with myocardial infarction. In contrast, patients with end-stage congestive heart failure demonstrate reduced LA contractile function. (Reprinted from *American Journal of Cardiology*, 81, Dernellis *et al*., Left atrial mechanical adaptation to long-standing hemodynamic loads based on pressure–volume relations, 1138–1143, Copyright 1998, with permission from Excerpta Medica [12].)

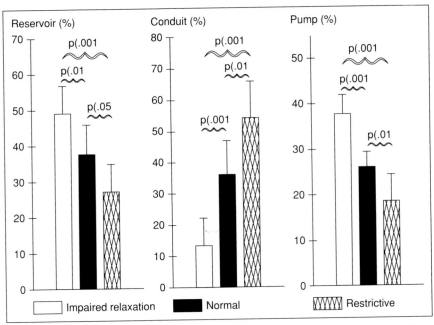

Fig. 3.7 Percent contribution to left ventricular (LV) filling of the left atrial (LA) reservoir, conduit and contractile function in relation to the different patterns of LV filling. Reservoir and pump function are significantly increased in patients with impaired relaxation compared with those with normal or restrictive patterns. In contrast, LA conduit function is augmented in patients with severe LV failure as LA contractile dysfunction occurs. (Reprinted from *American Journal of Cardiology*, 82, Prioli *et al.*, Increasing degrees of left ventricular filling impairment modulate left atrial function in humans, 756–761, Copyright 1998, with permission from Excerpta Medica [27].)

Atrial mechanics and arrhythmogenesis

Brief periods of AF ranging from minutes to hours cause reversible LA contractile dysfunction after restoration of sinus rhythm. Contractile dysfunction of LA stunned myocardium caused by brief AF is improved by the calcium (Ca^{2+}) channel blocker verapamil but worsened by the Ca^{2+} channel agonist Bay K 8644. These findings suggest that intracellular Ca^{2+} overload may be responsible for LA myocardial stunning [29]. However, the mechanism of atrial contractile dysfunction following AF may depend on the duration of the arrhythmia. Recently, Schotten and colleagues demonstrated that atrial contractile remodeling corresponds to electrical remodeling following AF of several days duration (Fig. 3.8) in chronically instrumented goats using sonomicrometer crystals to measure atrial dimension [30]. The L-type Ca^{2+} channel agonist Bay Y 5959 increased atrial contractility to the same extent as it prolonged the refractory period. These data indicate that both electrical and contractile remodeling result from similar cellular mechanisms, presumably related to intracellular Ca^{2+} handling. However, a separate mechanism may be responsible for longer-term loss of function despite recovery of atrial effective refractory period following prolonged duration AF.

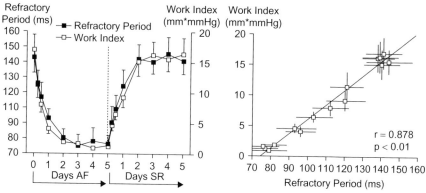

Fig. 3.8 Time course of atrial electrical and contractile remodeling, including reversibility (left). Right atrial work index is also correlated to the refractory period. Data are from seven chronically instrumented goats. (Reprinted from *Circulation*, 107, Schotten *et al.*, Electrical and contractile remodeling during the first days of atrial fibrillation go hand in hand, 1433–39, Copyright 2003, with permission from Lippincott, Williams and Wilkins [30].)

Atrial arrhythmias affect ventricular function. Chronic rapid atrial pacing produces a biatrial cardiomyopathy similar to that observed during AF [31], decreases the active contribution of the LA to LV filling, and eventually reduces the role of the LA to an inefficient conduit for PV blood flow [32]. Chronic LV hypovolemia, similar to that observed during severe mitral stenosis, also occurs, although cardiac output may be preserved by compensatory increases in sympathetic nervous system activity under these conditions. Recent clinical data suggest that the maintenance of sinus rhythm in patients with persistent AF by repeated cardioversion using an implantable device is associated with reversed remodeling of LV mechanical function [33, 34]. However, the overall role of reduced ventricular function secondary to atrial arrhythmias is still only partially understood.

Specific entities affecting left atrial mechanical function

Atrioventricular timing

Optimization of AV timing may enhance cardiac performance and may also prevent or attenuate the development of a pro-arrhythmic atrial substrate. As mentioned earlier, LA contractile function is associated with reductions in cardiac output when atrial contraction is inappropriately timed or eliminated [1, 25]. Skinner *et al.* [35] demonstrated the importance of AV timing in enhancing LV filling and reducing mitral valve regurgitation. The importance of the LA contribution to LV performance during ventricular pacing has also been shown [36]. Other clinical investigations have demonstrated an apparent advantage of atrial- relative to ventricular-based pacing in preventing the development of AF in patients requiring pacemakers with or without a history of atrial tachyarrhythmias. These studies suggest that single-chamber, right-ventricular apical pacing may lead to the development of AF by producing asynchronous ventricular depolarization and impairing LV efficiency [37]. These data also

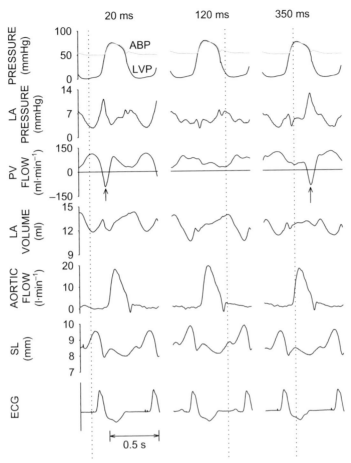

Fig. 3.9 Representative data from a dog with normal ventricular function during synchronous dual-chamber pacing from the right atrial appendage at three of six tested atrioventricular delays, including left ventricular (LVP), arterial (ABP) and left atrial (LA) pressures, pulmonary venous (PV) flow, left atrial volume (LAV), aortic blood flow, regional LV segment length (SL) and electrocardiogram (ECG). Programming the AV delay to 20 ms resulted in 'late' atrial depolarization and contraction after mitral valve closure. In contrast, LA contraction occurred during LV diastole and systole at AV delays of 120 and 350 ms, respectively. LV end-systolic pressure and peak aortic blood flow were greatest at an AV delay of 120 ms. Retrograde pulmonary venous blood flow was observed during LA contraction at AV delays of 20 and 350 (arrows) but not 120 ms. This retrograde flow corresponded with a premature decrease in LA volume during LV systole. Minimal LA volume was lowest and LV end-diastolic segment length was highest at an AV delay of 120 ms. Vertical dashed lines indicate timing of atrial pacing. (Reprinted from *PACE*, 25, Hettrick *et al.*, Effects of atrial pacing lead location and atrial–ventricular delay on atrial and ventricular hemodynamics in dogs, 888–96, Copyright 2002, with permission from Blackwell Publishing Ltd [7].)

emphasize the importance of maintaining the LA contribution to LV filling during right ventricular apical pacing. AV timing delay during dual chamber pacing affects PV flow, LA function and LV performance in anesthetized dogs with and without cardiomyopathy (Figs 3.9 and 3.10) [7, 8]. The importance of

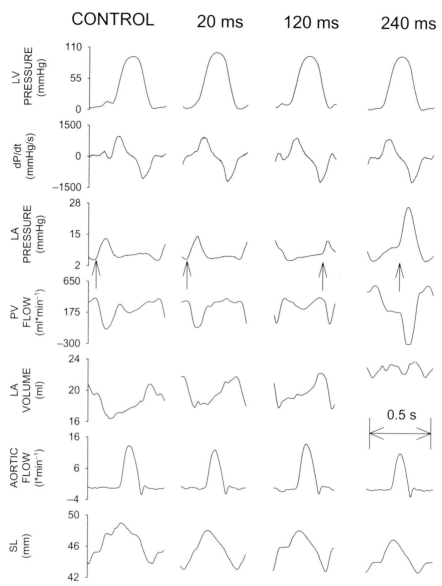

Fig. 3.10 Raw hemodynamic data from one dog with pacing-induced cardiomyopathy during normal sinus rhythm control and dual-chamber pacing from the left atrial lateral wall position with atrioventricular (AV) delays of 20, 120 and 240 ms at a heart rate of 120 b.p.m. Atrial contraction is associated with increased left atrial (LA) pressure and decreased pulmonary venous (PV) flow and atrial volume (arrow). Suboptimal AV delays (200 ms and 240 ms) result in larger deceleration of PV flow and smaller increases in LV diameter during atrial contraction. This results in decreased maximal aortic blood flow. (Reprinted from *PACE*, 26, Hettrick *et al.*, Atrial pacing lead location alters the hemodynamic effects of atrial–ventricular delay in heart failure, 853–61, Copyright 2003, with permission from Blackwell Publishing Ltd [8].)

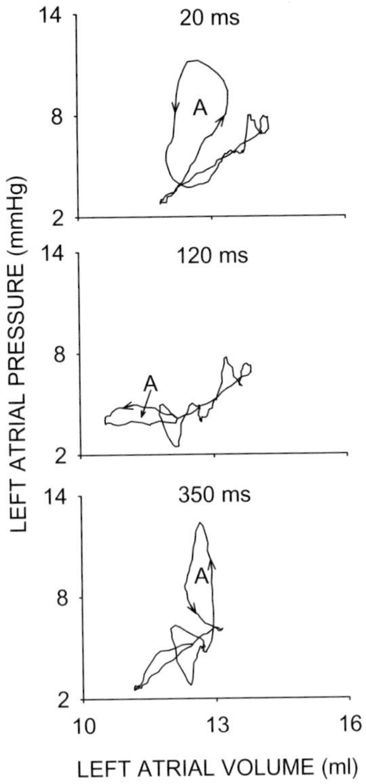

Fig. 3.11 Representative left atrial (LA) pressure–volume diagrams derived from the hemodynamic data in Fig. 3.8 during right atrial appendage pacing at three atrioventricular (AV) delays. Large, poorly synchronized 'a' loops occurred during pacing at AV delays of 20 and 350 ms because the LA contracts against a closed mitral valve (see text). (Reprinted from *PACE*, 25, Hettrick *et al.*, Effects of atrial pacing lead location and atrial–ventricular delay on atrial and ventricular hemodynamics in dogs, 888–96, Copyright 2002, with permission from Blackwell Publishing Ltd [7].)

AV timing delay in LA pressure–volume diagram morphology is illustrated in Figs 3.11 and 3.12. Large, poorly synchronized 'a' loops occur during pacing at AV delays of 20 and 350 ms because LA contraction occurs against a closed mitral valve. Increased LA stroke work then contributes to increases in retrograde PV flow rather than LV filling. Similar results have recently been demonstrated clinically in patients undergoing an electrophysiological procedure (Figs 3.13 and 3.14) [19]. In this study, right atrial pressure volume loops were measured using the conductance catheter technique [18]. Changes in both atrial and cardiovascular function (i.e. arterial pulse pressure; Fig. 3.14) were influenced by both atrial pacing lead location and AV delay. Thus, both laboratory and clinical data suggest that optimized AV timing may improve atrial efficiency and global cardiovascular function.

Inefficient atrial–ventricular mechanical coupling due to abnormal AV timing may affect atrial mechanical performance in several ways. First, increased atrial pressure leads to increased atrial wall stress. Such increases in stress produce corresponding increases in strain (manifested by atrial stretch), assuming constant atrial wall compliance [38]. However, if increased atrial myocardial stress is associated with increased atrial elastance (or stiffness), such as may occur during atrial systole (Figs 3.11, 3.12 and 3.13), then increased atrial stress may occur with minimal increased strain [7, 8, 19]. Finally, contraction of the

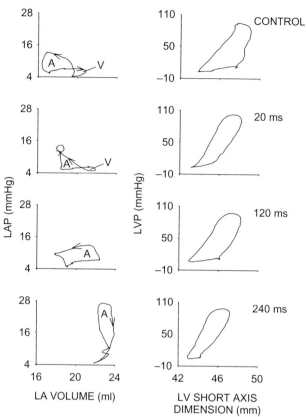

Fig. 3.12 Atrial (top) and ventricular (bottom) pressure–volume loops during normal sinus rhythm control and dual-chamber pacing from the left atrial lateral wall position with atrioventricular (AV) delays of 20, 120 and 240 ms at a heart rate of 120 b.p.m. Large increases in atrial pressure are not necessarily associated with proportionate increases in volume due to isovolumic atrial contraction. In this case, large 'a' waves represent increased atrial work but not increased filling, since the increased work results in retrograde pulmonary venous blood flow. The pressure–volume loops show the greatest stroke work when LA–AV coupling is maximized. (Reprinted from *PACE*, 26, Hettrick *et al.*, Atrial pacing lead location alters the hemodynamic effects of atrial–ventricular delay in heart failure, 853–61, Copyright 2003, with permission from Blackwell Publishing Ltd [8].)

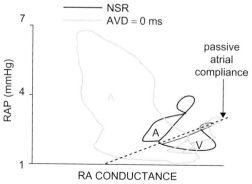

Fig. 3.13 Right atrial pressure–conductance loops from one patient with normal ventricular function during normal sinus rhythm and during dual-chamber pacing with an atrioventricular delay of 0 ms. Atrial contraction against a closed tricuspid valve results in isovolumic increase in atrial pressure. The increased 'a' loop area represents increased work performed by the atria, but not increased filling since the tricuspid valve is closed. Instead, retrograde perfusion of the vena cavae occurs.

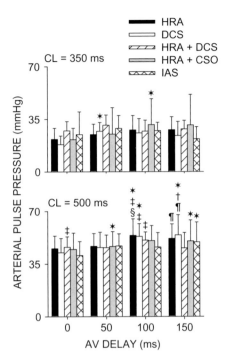

Fig. 3.14 Changes in arterial pulse pressure, an index of global ventricular performance, during single- and multisite pacing at various atrial sites, atrioventricular delays and two heart rates in patients ($n = 12$) with normal atrial and ventricular function. Pulse pressure was sensitive to both site and delay. *$P < 0.05$ versus 0 ms; †$P < 0.05$ versus 50 ms; ‡$P < 0.05$ versus IAS; §$P < 0.05$ versus HRA + CSO; ¶$P < 0.05$ versus HRA + DCS, ¶$P < 0.05$ versus HRA; $n = 12$. Data are mean ± SD. HRA = high right atrium; DCS = distal coronary sinus; CSO = coronary sinus ostium; IAS = inter-atrial septum.

atrium against a closed, or partially closed, tricuspid (or mitral) valve may lead to deceleration or frank reversal of caval (or pulmonary venous) flow, resulting in dramatic changes in the magnitude and direction of venous shear stress. The relative importance of changes in atrial wall stress, atrial wall strain, and venous shear stress (Figs 3.9 and 3.10) in the promotion of heterogeneous atrial substrate or in the exacerbation of atrial venous ectopic foci is unknown. However, it seems likely that such changes in shear stress patterns may be contributors to a pro-arrhythmic state. A recent study of biventricular pacing suggested that the functional benefits of improved LV contractile synchrony might be eliminated if AV timing is not optimized to facilitate LV filling [39]. Improvement of LA function using optimized AV delay may theoretically slow the progression of disease processes such as AF and heart failure by maintaining appropriate LA–LV coupling, reducing retrograde PV blood flow and preventing the development of the pro-arrhythmic atrial substrate necessary to sustain AF. Future clinical studies of the influence of alternate site atrial pacing and AV delay on atrioventricular mechanical coupling relationships should focus on pressure volume analysis of both chambers (Fig. 3.15) and the ratio of atrial systolic elastance to ventricular diastolic elastance [15].

Appendage resection

The atrial appendage may contribute to the ability of the atrial myocardium to store a substantial volume of blood at low energy cost (i.e. reservoir function).

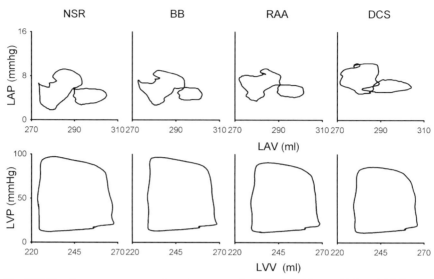

Fig. 3.15 Simultaneous pressure–volume loops recorded in the left atrium and left ventricle in an anesthetized pig using the conductance catheter technique during normal sinus rhythm (NSR) and during dual-chamber pacing from different atrial lead locations, including the high right atrial septum (Bachmann's bundle region; BB), right atrial appendage (RAA) and distal coronary sinus (DCS) at similar atrioventricular delays (100 ms). Note that raw data are not adjusted for parallel conductance volume. These data demonstrate the subtle effects of alternate atrial pacing lead locations on atrial performance, ventricular performance and atrioventricular mechanical coupling relationships. Optimized lead location and atrioventricular timing may lead to improved cardiovascular performance.

Thus, the atrial appendages serve as dedicated compliance chambers with important roles in preserving LA compliance. Clamping or excision of the LA appendage [26, 40] adversely affects LA reservoir function and reduces left atrial compliance. Novel catheter-based techniques designed to isolate the left atrial appendage have been used recently to decrease the risk of embolic stroke, but whether such LA appendage isolation adversely affects reservoir function in a similar fashion remains unknown. Given the experimental data indicating the importance of the LA compliance, however, further clinical study of the pathophysiologic affects of LA appendage isolation are warranted.

Ablation

Traditional surgical and catheter Maze procedures, as well as evolving techniques for pulmonary venous isolation, result in significant compartmentalization of the atria. These procedures may also result in loss of tissue or 'debulking'. It is reasonable to hypothesize that altered contractile patterns of the atria and the loss of compliant tissue may result in substantial alteration in atrial mechanical function after ablation. Conversely, patients undergoing these procedures typically present with severely dilated atria and profoundly depressed atrial function that may be improved by a reduction in chamber size. An acute

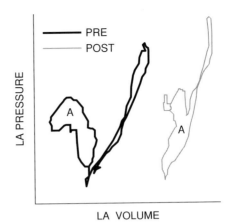

Fig. 3.16 Left atrial pressure–conductance volume diagrams from an individual patient before versus after radiofrequency ablation involving complete isolation of myocardium included proximal to right and left pulmonary venous inflow vestibules.

investigation of atrial function before compared with after ablation revealed no changes in atrial pressure, atrial systolic function or atrial reservoir function immediately after PV isolation (Fig. 3.16). No significant difference was observed in 'a' loop area before compared with after isolation (48 ± 25 versus 49 ± 31 mmHg/ml, $P > 0.005$, $n = 15$). These data were obtained using a combination conductance–pressure catheter introduced into the LA via a trans-septal venous approach. However, few data currently exist to examine the acute and long-term effects of atrial ablation procedures on atrial conduit, reservoir and pump function.

References

1 Barbier P, Solomon SB, Schiller NB, Glantz SA. Left atrial relaxation and left ventricular systolic function determine left atrial reservoir function. *Circulation* 1999; **100**: 427–36.

2 Li D, Fareh S, Leung TK, Nattel S. Promotion of atrial fibrillation by heart failure in dogs – atrial remodeling of a different kind. *Circulation* 1999; **100**: 87–95.

3 Lakatta EG, Levy D. Arterial and cardiac aging: major shareholders in cardiovascular disease enterprises. Part I. Aging arteries: a 'set up' for vascular disease. *Circulation* 2003; **107**: 139–46.

4 Lakatta EG, Levy D. Arterial and cardiac aging: major shareholders in cardiovascular disease enterprises. Part II. The aging heart in health: links to heart disease. *Circulation* 2003; **107**: 346–54.

5 Mitchell JH, Shapiro W. Atrial function and the hemodynamic consequences of atrial fibrillation in man. *Am J Cardiol* 1969; **23**: 556–67.

6 Miyaguchi K, Iwase M, Matsui H *et al.* Role of left atrial booster pump function in a worsening course of congestive heart failure. *Jpn Circ J* 1992; **56**: 509–17.

7 Hettrick DA, Euler DE, Pagel PS *et al.* Effects of atrial pacing lead location and atrial–ventricular delay on atrial and ventricular hemodynamics in dogs. *Pacing Clin Electrophysiol* 2002; **25**: 888–96.

8 Hettrick, DA, Warltier DC, Tessmer JH *et al.* Atrial pacing lead location alters the hemodynamic effects of atrial–ventricular delay in heart failure. *Pacing Clin Electrophysiol* 2003; **26**: 853–61.

9   Little RC. Volume pressure relationships of the pulmonary-left heart vascular segment. Evidence for a 'valve-like' closure of the pulmonary veins. *Circ Res* 1960; **8**: 594–9.

10 Alexander J, Sunagawa K, Chang N, Sagawa K. Instantaneous pressure–volume relation of the ejecting canine left atrium. *Circ Res* 1987; **61**: 209–19.

11 Oki T, Tabata T, Yamada H, Fukuda K *et al*. Assessment of abnormal left atrial relaxation by transesopheal pulsed Doppler echocardiography of pulmonary venous flow velocity. *Clin Cardiol* 1998; **21**: 753–8.

12 Dernellis JM, Stefanadis CI, Zacharoulis AA, Toutouzas PK. Left atrial mechanical adaptation to long-standing hemodynamic loads based on pressure–volume relations. *Am J Cardiol* 1998; **81**: 1138–43.

13 Hoit BD, Shao Y, Gabel M, Walsh RA. In vivo assessment of left atrial contractile performance in normal and pathological conditions using a time-varying elastance model. *Circulation* 1994; **89**: 1829–38.

14 Daoud EG, Marcovitz P, Knight BP *et al*. Short-term effect of atrial fibrillation on atrial contractile function in humans. *Circulation* 1999; **99**: 3024–7.

15 Suga H. Importance of atrial compliance in cardiac performance. *Circ Res* 1974; **35**: 39–43.

16 Nagano R, Masuyama T, Naka M, Hori M, Kamada T. Contribution of atrial reservoir function to ventricular filling in hypertensive patients. Effects of nifedipine administration. *Hypertension* 1995; **26**: 815–19.

17 Tabata T, Oki T, Yamada H *et al*. Role of left atrial appendage in left atrial reservoir function as evaluated by left atrial appendage clamping during cardiac surgery. *Am J Cardiol* 1998; **81**: 327–32.

18 Ferguson JJ, Miller MJ, Aroesty JM *et al*. Assessment of right atrial pressure–volume relations in patients with and without atrial septal defect. *J Am Coll Cardiol* 1989; **13**: 630–6.

19 Tse HF, Lau CP, Hettrick DA. Single and dual site atrial lead location alter the acute hemodynamic response to atrial–ventricular delay [abstract]. *J Am Coll Cardiol* 2002; **39**: 86A.

20 Mohan JC, Arora R. Effects of atrial fibrillation on left ventricular function and geometry in mitral stenosis. *Am J Cardiol* 1997; **80**: 1618–20.

21 Kono T, Sabbah HN, Rosman H *et al*. Left atrial contribution to ventricular filling during the course of evolving heart failure. *Circulation* 1992; **86**: 1317–22.

22 Matsuzaki M, Tanitani M, Toma Y *et al*. Mechanism of augmented left atrial pump function in myocardial infarction and essential hypertension evaluated by left atrial pressure dimension relation. *Am J Cardiol* 1991; **67**: 1121–6.

23 Panagiotopoulos K, Toumanidis S, Saridakis N, Vemmos K, Moulopoulos S. Left atrial and left atrial appendage functional abnormalities in patients with cardioembolic stroke in sinus rhythm and idiopathic atrial fibrillation. *J Am Soc Echocardiogr* 1998; **11**: 711–19.

24 Leistad E, Christensen G, Ilebekk A. Effects of atrial fibrillation on left and right atrial dimensions, pressures, and compliances. *Am J Physiol Heart Circ Physiol* 1993; **264**: H1093–7.

25 Hoit BD, Shao Y, Gabel M. Left atrial systolic and diastolic function accompanying chronic rapid pacing-induced atrial failure. *Am J Physiol Heart Circ Physiol* 1998; **275**: H183–9.

26 Hoit BD, Shao Y, Tsai LM *et al*. Altered left atrial compliance after atrial appendectomy. Influence on left atrial and ventricular filling. *Circ Res* 1993; **72**: 167–75.

27 Prioli A, Marino P, Lanzoni L, Zardini P. Increasing degrees of left ventricular filling impairment modulate left atrial function in humans. *Am J Cardiol* 1998; **82**: 756–61.

28 Ritter O, Luther HP, Haase H *et al*. Expression of atrial myosin light chains but not alpha-myosin heavy chains is correlated in vivo with increased ventricular function in patients with hypertrophic obstructive cardiomyopathy. *J Mol Med* 1999; **77**: 677–85.

29 Leistad E, Aksnes G, Verburg E, Christensen G. Atrial contractile dysfunction after short-term atrial fibrillation is reduced by verapamil but increased by BAY K8644. *Circulation* 1996; **93**: 1747–54.

30 Schotten U, Duytschaever M, Ausma J, Eijsbouts S, Neuberger HR, Allessie M. Electrical and contractile remodeling during the first days of atrial fibrillation go hand in hand. *Circulation* 2003; **107**: 1433–9.

31 Zipes DP. Atrial fibrillation. A tachycardia-induced atrial cardiomyopathy. *Circulation* 1997; **95**: 562–4.

32 Hoit BD, Shao Y, Gabel M. Global and regional atrial function after rapid atrial pacing: an echo doppler study. *J Am Soc Echocardiogr* 1997; **10**: 805–10.

33 Tse HF, Lau CP, Yu CM *et al*. Effect of the implantable atrial defibrillator on the natural history of atrial fibrillation. *J Cardiovasc Electrophysiol* 1999; **10**: 1200–9.

34 Tse HF, Wang Q, Yu CM, Ayers GM, Lau CP. Time course of recovery of left atrial mechanical dysfunction after cardioversion of spontaneous atrial fibrillation with the implantable atrial defibrillator. *Am J Cardiol* 2000; **86**: 1023–5.

35 Skinner NS, Mitchell JH, Wallace AG, Sarnoff SJ. Hemodynamic effects of altering the timing of atrial systole. *Am J Physiol* 1963; **205**: 499–503.

36 Ruskin J, McHale PA, Harley A, Greenfield JC Jr. Pressure-flow studies in man: effect of atrial systole on left ventricular function. *J Clin Invest* 1970; **49**: 472–8.

37 Yamamoto K, Kodama K, Masuyama T *et al*. Role of atrial contraction and synchrony of ventricular contraction in the optimisation of ventriculoarterial coupling in humans. *Br Heart J* 1992; **67**: 361–7.

38 Bode F, Katchman A, Woosley RL, Franz MR. Gadolinium decreases stretch-induced vulnerability to atrial fibrillation. *Circulation* 2000; **101**: 2200–5.

39 Saxon LA, Hourigan L, Guerra P *et al*. Influence of programmed AV delay on left ventricular performance in biventricular pacing systems for the treatment of heart failure. *J Am Coll Cardiol* 2000; **35**: 166A.

40 Ito T, Suwa M, Hirota Y *et al*. Influence of left atrial function on Doppler transmitral and pulmonary venous flow patterns in dilated and hypertrophic cardiomyopathy: evaluation of left atrial appendage function by transesophageal echocardiography. *Am Heart J* 1996; **131**: 122–30.

CHAPTER 4

Molecular Basis of Atrial Fibrillation

Samir Saba, Barry London

Since the first success of transgenesis and gene targeting in the early 1980s [1–3], advances in molecular genetics have transformed cardiovascular medical research. Significant progress came with the introduction of homologous recombinant technology [3], which has allowed the manipulation of the mammalian genome with great precision by introducing targeted mutations at specific DNA sequences, causing the elimination or modification of specific gene products. Additional advances have included conditional, tissue-specific gene-targeted mutations and inducible transgenic manipulations [4]. These techniques made possible the creation of animal models of cardiac diseases in which the genetic defect is accurately defined and carried over the animal's lifetime and transmitted through the germ line.

Of all the candidate animals for genetic engineering, the mouse has quickly become the most attractive, given the genetic, technical and economic advantages that it offers [5, 6]. For the physiologist, however, its small size and extremely short cardiac cycle length (one-tenth of that of humans) present technical challenges to the extraction of meaningful phenotypic information about the function of the targeted gene. Adapting the tools of clinical cardiac diagnosis (echocardiography, magnetic resonance imaging, invasive and non-invasive hemodynamic and electrophysiological testing, etc.) to the murine anatomy and physiology has therefore become of utmost importance in overcoming this problem.

As the molecular basis of an expanding spectrum of cardiovascular diseases associated with arrhythmias and conduction abnormalities is being revealed [7, 8] and mouse models are being created for them, invasive electrophysiological techniques are developing. Examples of transgenic strains with a bearing on cardiac electrophysiology include models of gap junction protein deficiency (connexins 40, 43, and 45), ion channel deficiency or overexpression, hypertrophic cardiomyopathy, and long-QT syndrome.

Atrial fibrillation (AF) is the most common sustained clinical arrhythmia, with a prevalence of about 1% in the general population of the USA and close to 10% in patients older than 70 years [9]. It is also one of the leading causes of thromboembolism, accounting for about 75 000 strokes every year [10]. Although AF cases are primarily sporadic and associated with risk factors such as valvular heart disease and hypertension, familial cases of AF have been described [11–13]. Most of the genetic abnormalities in the familial form of AF have not yet been elucidated, but reports have described loci on chromosome 10 (10q22–q24) and chromosome 6 (6q14–16) [14, 15]. In addition, a missense mutation in the K+ channel KCNQ1 (KvLQT1) that is responsible for the slowly activating delayed rectifier current I_{Ks} causes AF in one family [16]. Other reports have implicated the 38G polymorphism of the minK gene, alterations in the L-type calcium current, and/or a number of other potassium currents (minK, Kv4.3, Kv1.5, HERG and Kir3.1) in the initiation or maintenance of AF [17, 18]. Even though AF is primarily an acquired disorder, the insights gained from studying the familial forms of the disease can greatly improve the understanding of the pathogenesis of AF and eventually affect the way it is treated or prevented. For now, however, the molecular pathways leading to AF in most affected patients remain poorly understood.

This chapter will review the techniques used to engineer transgenic and gene-targeted mice, the various techniques used in murine electrophysiological testing, and the transgenic and wild-type mouse models of AF described in the literature. We believe that the mouse can be a valuable animal model for uncovering the genetic and molecular bases of human AF.

Methods for engineering transgenic and gene-targeted mice

Transgenic overexpression

Transgenic mice are most commonly used to study the effects of overexpression of a gene in the heart (Fig. 4.1A). The transgenic construct comprises the promoter that directs the age and tissue-specificity of expression, the transgene to be expressed, and a poly-A tail to stabilize the RNA. The transgenic construct is injected directly into the pronucleus of a fertilized mouse oocyte, which is then implanted into a pseudopregnant female. Founders (F_0 generation) are identified by screening DNA obtained from tail biopsies of live offspring using PCR or genomic Southern blots and mated with wild-type mice to generate heterozygous F_1 offspring. The F_1 mice are then examined for transgene expression. Using this method, littermate controls are readily available and studies may be completed in as little as 1 year. In addition, overexpression of inhibitory or dominant negative constructs can be used to decrease the expression of genes using this strategy [19].

The most common promoter used for cardiovascular studies was derived from the rat or mouse α-myosin heavy chain gene, because it becomes active near birth (avoiding problems associated with embryonic lethality) and directs expression of the transgene specifically to the ventricles and atria of the adult mouse [20]. One difficulty with mice using this promoter relates to uncertainty about whether the effects in the atria are due to direct expression of the transgene in atrial myocytes or whether they are indirect effects due to expression in the ventricles. Promoters that express specifically in the atrium [e.g. the atrial natriuretic factor (ANF) promoter] would circumvent this difficulty [21]. Of note, transgenic mice have not typically been engineered specifically for the purpose of studying atrial arrhythmias.

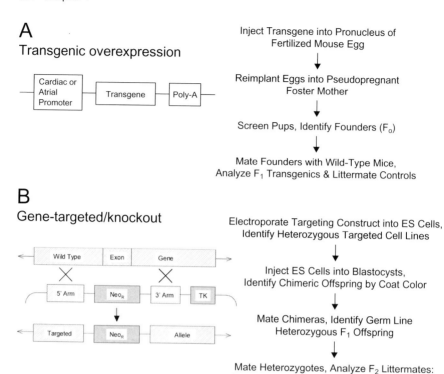

A

Transgenic overexpression

Inject Transgene into Pronucleus of Fertilized Mouse Egg

↓

Reimplant Eggs into Pseudopregnant Foster Mother

↓

Screen Pups, Identify Founders (F_0)

↓

Mate Founders with Wild-Type Mice, Analyze F_1 Transgenics & Littermate Controls

B

Gene-targeted/knockout

Electroporate Targeting Construct into ES Cells, Identify Heterozygous Targeted Cell Lines

↓

Inject ES Cells into Blastocysts, Identify Chimeric Offspring by Coat Color

↓

Mate Chimeras, Identify Germ Line Heterozygous F_1 Offspring

↓

Mate Heterozygotes, Analyze F_2 Littermates: Homozygotes, Heterozygotes, and Wild Type

Fig. 4.1 Comparison of the techniques used to engineer transgenic mice and gene-targeted knockout mice. (A) The transgenic construct (left) randomly inserts into the chromosome. Note that experimental mice are available after only two breeding cycles. (B) The knockout construct (left) is electroporated into mouse embryonic stem cells that are then used to engineer mice. Homologous recombination, or a double crossover event, is denoted by X. Note that at least three breeding cycles are required to obtain experimental animals, and that only one-quarter of the F_2 mice will be homozygotes. Neo_R = neomycin resistance gene; TK = thymidine kinase gene.

Random incorporation of the transgene into a mouse chromosome may disrupt the function of a native gene at the insertion site. Another potential problem with transgenic mice arises from the massive overexpression of a mutant protein. The protein may titrate away important factors or have direct toxic effects on cardiac myocytes, as illustrated by the dilated cardiomyopathy caused by overexpression of green fluorescent protein [22]. Ideally, transgene expression in the heart could be turned on and off at will. A number of systems have been developed, some based on the use of tetracycline-responsive promoter elements [23]. These systems require the mating of two transgenic mice, one with the transgene of interest driven by a ubiquitous promoter engineered to require a specific DNA-binding protein for activity and the other with a tissue-specific promoter driving the drug-responsive DNA binding protein. To date, limited success rates and variable tissue specificity of the transgene (leakiness) have prevented widespread use of this technology. To our knowledge, no transgenic mice with inducible atrial expression have been reported.

Gene targeting

Individual genes can be inactivated (gene knockout) or modified (gene knockin, targeted mutagenesis) in the mouse using homologous recombination in embryonic stem (ES) cells (Fig. 4.1B) [4]. ES cells are produced from the inner cell mass of male blastocysts and expanded *in vitro*, and are unique in that they maintain the ability to differentiate into all cell types including germ cells. The cells used most frequently were produced from SV129 mice that are homozygous for a dominant gene that codes for the agouti coat color. DNA from the gene of interest is cloned, a targeting construct is engineered, and is then introduced into ES cells by electroporation (electric shock). A small fraction of the cells undergo homologous recombination, whereby two cross-over events replace the portion of the gene between the homologous arms of the targeting construct with an antibiotic resistance cassette and any other DNA in the targeting construct. This results in a small number of ES cells heterozygous for the targeted allele. Heterozygous ES cells are then injected into blastocysts harvested from C57BL/6 mice with black coat color, and implanted into pseudopregnant females. Chimeric offspring, in part derived from ES cells and in part from the donor blastocysts, are identified by their mixed agouti/black coat color. The male chimeras are mated with female C57BL/6 mice and germline transmission of ES cell-derived sperm is determined by the agouti coat color of the offspring. Half of these agouti offspring carry one copy of the targeted allele. Heterozygous male and female mice are mated to each other to yield homozygous targeted mice.

This form of gene manipulation has several important sequelae. The targeted allele is present in all cell types in which the gene is expressed. Consequently, any phenotype reflects the loss of the gene not only from the heart but also from the nervous system and potentially other tissues. In addition, the targeted allele is present throughout embryonic development. As a result, the phenotype of the adult mouse may be modified by long-term compensatory changes in other genes, and embryonic lethality may preclude the study of the role of some genes in the adult mouse. In addition, the strain of the mouse can affect the phenotype produced by the genetic manipulations.

The ability to engineer gene knockouts in a time- and tissue-restricted manner has been developed using the cre/lox system. Here, gene targeting is used to surround the desired gene by two 34-bp loxP elements. Homozygous targeted mice are then mated with transgenic mice that express the cre recombinase enzyme in a tissue- and time-specific manner. In the presence of the cre recombinase protein, the part of gene between the loxP elements is removed and the conditional tissue-specific knockout completed. As with transgenic mice, a promoter could be used to drive cre expression specifically in the atrium.

Electrophysiologic testing in the mouse

Ex vivo electrophysiological testing in the mouse

Isolated perfused heart models provide the physiologists with the ability to study the heart as an isolated organ, without the influence of the autonomic nervous system. It also permits the fine regulation of its immediate milieu in terms of its composition, pH, temperature, oxygen content and drug concentration, simply by modifying the composition of the perfusate that is being provided by the Langendorff apparatus. This technique has been widely used

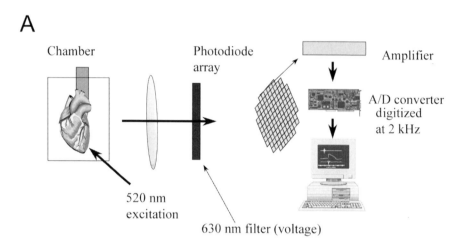

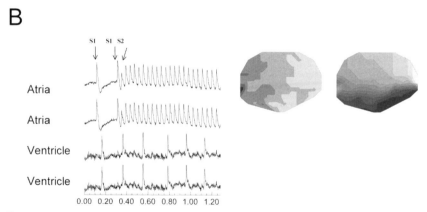

Fig. 4.2 Optical mapping of murine action potentials in Langendorff-perfused mouse hearts. (A) Schematic representation of the optical mapping setup for use with the mouse. The fluorescent signal from a 4 x 4 mm region of the epicardial surface of the mouse heart is focused on a 124 element photodiode array, yielding 124 simultaneous action potentials signals. (B) Induction of atrial flutter (rate ~1400 beats/minute) by a single premature atrial stimulus in a TNF-α transgenic heart. Note that the top two channels are recording atrial action potentials, while the bottom two are recording intermittent ventricular activation.

in various animal models, including the mouse [24–27]. At our institution, this technique has been coupled with programmed stimulation and high-resolution optical mapping (voltage- and calcium-sensitive dyes) to study the characteristics of impulse propagation, conduction velocities and arrhythmo-genesis of various mouse models [28, 29]. We have recently adapted these techniques for the atrium (Fig. 4.2).

Electrocardiograms and ambulatory monitoring

As in humans, electrocardiograms can be performed on mice. Because of their small size and rapid heart rates, care must be taken to optimize lead contact and avoid overfiltering of the signal. This often requires subcutaneous electrodes and anesthetics that can alter heart rate and/or AV nodal function. Implant-able wireless radiofrequency transmitters (DataSciences International, St Paul, Minnesota, USA) have been inserted in mice for continuous ambulatory monitor-ing of cardiac rate and rhythm [30, 31]. A few days after surgery, the mouse is placed in its cage over a receiver plate. The single-lead electrocardiogram is then digitized and saved on a computer for analysis. Using this technique, quantification arrhythmia and analysis of heart rate variability can be performed on ambulatory mice without anesthesia (Fig. 4.3A). Evaluation of the effect of drugs on cardiac rhythm can also be achieved using this technique [32].

In vivo electrophysiological testing in the mouse

Whole-animal preparations have been widely used in large animals to study the properties of cardiac conduction [33, 34]. With the mouse rapidly evolving into the principal mammalian species for transgenic studies, an *in vivo* approach to mouse electrophysiological testing was developed [35]. This novel technique in its earliest phases adopted an open-chest approach but was soon replaced by an endovascular technique using a 1.7 French octapolar catheter (NuMed, Hopkinton, New York, USA), which is less invasive, technic-ally simpler, and allows the recording of a His-bundle electrogram [36, 37]. With this technique, complete *in vivo* electrophysiological testing became feasible in the mouse, similarly to what is done in humans and large mammals (Fig. 4.3B).

Mouse models of atrial fibrillation

Induced (non-transgenic)

Large animal models that initiate and sustain AF include the dog [38], the goat [39], the pig [40] and others. These models have utilized various techniques, ranging from anatomical injuries to the atria, sterile pericarditis, rapid atrial or ventricular pacing with or without mitral regurgitation, vagal nerve stimula-tion and an assortment of chemical substances, such as cesium chloride and ethanol [41]. In wild-type mice, models of AF have been very rare owing to the small size of the murine heart and atria (100 mg and 7 mg, respectively) and the limited mass necessary to sustain a micro-re-entrant rhythm such as AF.

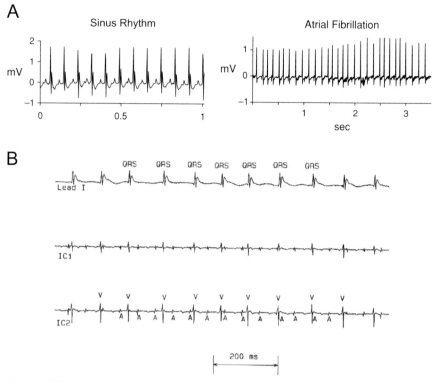

Fig. 4.3 (A) Electrocardiograms from a control mouse in sinus rhythm (left) and a TNF-α transgenic mouse with atrial fibrillation/flutter (right). Note that P-waves are not seen in the TNF-α mouse. (B) Atrial re-entrant tachycardia at a cycle length of 54 ms, with variable atrioventricular conduction, induced by a single atrial extrastimulus in a TNF-α mouse. The upper tracing represents lead I on the surface electrocardiogram. The second and third tracings represent intracardiac (IC_1 and IC_2) electrograms. A = atrial intracardiac deflection; V = ventricular intracardiac deflection; QRS = QRS complex on the surface ECG.

Despite these limitations, attempts have continued to create, induce and sustain AF in mice. Wakimoto *et al.* were able to induce AF in anesthetized wild-type C57BL6 mice by rapid endocardial atrial pacing [42]. Fourteen such mice underwent *in vivo*, closed-chest electrophysiological testing at baseline and after the intraperitoneal administration of carbamyl choline (50 ng/g) for cholinergic stimulation. At baseline, AF was inducible with atrial premature or burst pacing in one of 14 mice, compared with 11 out of 14 after carbamyl choline injection. The stimulation protocol included up to three premature extra-stimuli at a cycle length of 150 ms down to a minimum coupling interval of 10 ms or burst pacing with eight beats at a cycle length of 50 ms or four beats at 30 ms. The total duration of the stimulation protocol was limited to 1 minute. The mean duration of AF induced with this technique was 126 seconds, the longest episode (terminated with atropine) lasting 35 minutes. Schrickel *et al.* described a similar model of AF but with atrial pacing delivered through the transesophageal route [43]. In 40 C57BL6 wild-type mice (19 females), AF was induced by rapid atrial pacing at a mean cycle length of 27.4 ms in 36 (90%) of the animals. The four non-inducible mice were all females. In this study, AF was sustained for a mean duration of about 27 seconds before spontaneous termination. No pharmacological intervention aside from anesthesia was used to help induce or sustain the atrial arrhythmia in this model. Other scarce reports describe the use of $CaCl_2$–acetylcholine in conjunction with escalating doses of aconitine, ouabain or adrenaline to induce AF in murine hearts [44, 45]. These reports describe a protective role of cycloprotobuxine-A and cycloprotobuxine-D against the induction of AF.

Transgenic

A few transgenic mouse models exhibiting AF or atrial flutter have been described in the literature (Table 4.1). Most, but not all of them exhibit atrial arrhythmias in the context of a structural cardiac abnormality such as heart failure, atrial dilatation, or fibrosis. The following is a review of the most prominent of the murine transgenic models of AF.

Connexin-deficient mice

Connexins (Cx) are proteins that provide the building blocks for the gap junctions, which are bridges that facilitate electrical and ionic propagation between adjacent cells [46]. There are three main types of connexins expressed in the mammalian heart: Cx43 is present in both the atria and the ventricles; Cx40 is primarily present in the atria and the atrioventricular conduction system; and Cx45 is probably present in the atria but at lower levels. Knockout mouse models of these three types of Cx have been engineered. The homozygous knockout of Cx43 (Cx43$^{-/-}$) and Cx45 (Cx45$^{-/-}$) mice are not compatible with life [47–49]. Heterozygous Cx43$^{+/-}$ mice have normal cardiac development but

Table 4.1 Transgenic and gene-targeted mouse models of atrial fibrillation

Mouse model	Gene	Rhythm disturbances	Reference
Gap junction protein KO	Connexin40	AF (I); AV block	50
Ion channel KO	GIRK4	Protection against AF	56
Structural protein overexpression TG	Junctin	AF (S)	57
Metabolic protein overexpression TG	PAHX-AP1	AF (isolated atria)	59
Cytokine overexpression TG	TNF-α	AF (S, I), VA	28
Transcription factor and signaling molecule overexpression TGs	TGF-β1	AF (I)	66
	RhoA	AF (S), AV block	67
	RTEF	AF (S, I), AV block	69

KO = knockout, targeted disruption; TG = transgenic; AF = atrial fibrillation; I = inducible; S = spontaneous; AV = atrioventricular; VA = ventricular arrhythmia.

delayed ventricular conduction, although the results of the studies are some-
what controversial and method-dependent. A conditional knockout mouse
lacking Cx43 has marked impairment of ventricular conduction and dies of
ventricular fibrillation [47]. Homozygous ($Cx40^{-/-}$) and heterozygous ($Cx40^{+/-}$)
Cx40-deficient mice have been studied extensively from the electrophysiological standpoint. Hagendorff *et al.* studied these mice by subjecting them
to rapid transesophageal atrial pacing [50]. They documented a significant
increase in the sinus node recovery time, atrioventricular nodal Wenckebach
periodicity, and the intra-atrial conduction time in the $Cx40^{-/-}$ mice compared
with the $Cx40^{+/-}$ and $Cx40^{+/+}$ mice, implicating Cx40 in sinus node function and
atrioventricular conduction. More importantly, $Cx40^{-/-}$ mice, unlike their heterozygous and wild-type counterparts, had easily inducible atrial arrhythmias
(five out of eight mice) with burst atrial pacing. These atrial arrhythmias were
for the most part irregular and suggestive of AF. All episodes of AF were self-
terminated. Verheule *et al.* compared the electrophysiological characteristics
of $Cx40^{-/-}$ and $Cx40^{+/-}$ mice, using an open-chest epicardial technique [51].
Consistently with the study by Hagendorff *et al.*, the sinus node recovery time
and atrioventricular nodal Wenckebach periodicity were prolonged in the
knockout compared with the wild-type mice. Here also, burst atrial pacing
induced atrial arrhythmias in five out of ten $Cx40^{-/-}$ mice and in none of the
nine $Cx40^{+/+}$ mice. Heterozygous $Cx40^{+/-}$ mice did not differ from the $Cx40^{+/+}$
mice in any respect. We conducted a similar study in Cx40-deficient mice
using a closed-chest endocardial approach [52]. Our findings were similar
to the results of the two other studies. Moreover, we demonstrated that the
$Cx40^{-/-}$ mice exhibit conduction delays both at the level of the atrioventricular
node and in the His–Purkinje system. Based on these studies, Cx40 deficiency
in the mouse heart seems to increase the vulnerability of the heart to AF. Of
note, low levels of Cx40 adjusted to levels of Cx43 were documented in the
hearts of goats with AF induced by rapid atrial pacing [53]. This shows that
conditions that induce AF may lead to changes in gene expression that propagate the arrhythmic phenotype.

GIRK4 knockout mice

High vagal tone has been associated with the initiation of paroxysmal AF in
humans [54]. In mice, pretreatment of wild-type mice with carbamyl choline
increases the inducibility of AF with rapid atrial pacing [42]. GIRK1 and GIRK4
are two subunits required for the muscarinic-gated potassium channel I_{KACh}.
In the absence of GIRK4, GIRK1 does not form an active ionic channel and this
results in the elimination of I_{KACh}. In mammals, this current is present in the sinus
node, atrial tissue, atrioventricular node and His–Purkinje system [55]. I_{KACh}
mediates most of the vagal response in cardiac tissue. Kovoor *et al.* reported
protection against AF based on deficiency in the GIRK4 gene. Wild-type and
I_{KACh}-deficient mice underwent *in vivo* electrophysiological testing before and
after intraperitoneal injections of the muscarinic receptor agonist carbachol [56].
In the presence of carbachol, ten out of 14 wild-type mice were inducible for

AF. The episodes lasted an average of 5.7 minutes. No animals were induced into AF prior to carbachol administration. None of the I_{KACh}–deficient mice were inducible into AF despite the use of carbachol. Thus, this gene-targeted mouse model is protective against vagally mediated vulnerability to AF.

Junctin overexpression mice

Junctin is a major transmembrane protein in cardiac junctional sarcoplasmic reticulum, and forms a quaternary complex together with the ryanodine receptor, triadin and calsequestrin. Transgenic mice overexpressing canine junctin have been shown to exhibit cardiac hypertrophy (the heart-to-body weight ratio increasing approximately two-fold), impaired relaxation and increased atrial fibrosis [57, 58]. Compared with wild-type mice, transgenic mice overexpressing junctin have a significantly lower heart rate and evidence of AF on surface electrocardiograms, with the absence of P waves and irregular QRS complexes. No further electrophysiological characterization of this transgenic model is available.

PAHX-AP1 overexpression mice

Refsum disease is an autosomal recessive disorder of lipid metabolism. Its cardiac manifestations include tachycardia, dilatation and valvular abnormalities. Targeted cardiac overexpression of the Refsum disease gene-associated protein (PAHX-AP1) was engineered in mice under the control of the α-myosin heavy chain promoter [59]. In the transgenic mice, PAHX-AP1 overexpression, primarily in the right atrium and sinus node, led to higher heart rates under anesthesia, using surface electrocardiography. In isolated atria, atrial arrhythmias were induced by aconitine, a known inhibitor of sodium channel inactivation. The inducibility of atrial arrhythmias in this model has not been demonstrated *in vivo*. Of interest, targeted disruption of the genes SCP2 and SCPx inhibits branch-chain fatty acid metabolism (similar to Refsum disease) and leads to bradyarrhythmias when mice are fed a diet enriched in phytol [60].

TNF-α overexpression mice

AF is a common arrhythmia in patients with left ventricular dysfunction and is associated with increased morbidity and mortality [61]. The failing heart expresses the inflammatory cytokine tumor necrosis factor-α (TNF-α). Kubota *et al.* described a mouse model of non-ischemic cardiomyopathy and heart failure, based on targeted overexpression of TNF-α in the heart [62]. The transgenic mice exhibit heart failure signs, with increased heart-to-body weight ratio, cardiac chamber dilatation and reduced ejection fraction. Mice overexpressing TNF-α also exhibit sex-related survival differences that could be related to differential expression of myocardial TNF receptors [63]. From the electrophysiological perspective, the transgenic hearts are susceptible to re-entrant ventricular arrhythmias, as documented *in vitro* (12 out of 13 transgenic hearts versus no control hearts with inducible ventricular tachycardia) [28]. The mice overexpressing TNF-α were more likely to be inducible into atrial flutter with premature atrial stimulation during *in vivo* closed-chest electro-physiological testing. Here again, there were gender differences in the vulnerability of the transgenic mice to atrial arrhythmias, with a greater incidence of AF in males. Our data also show that the transgenic hearts are more vulnerable to atrial flutter *in vitro*, where single premature atrial stimuli elicited slow atrial conduction and re-entrant atrial tachycardias at rates up to 1500 beats/minute in six out of six TNF-α transgenic but in none of four control hearts.

TGF-β1 overexpression mice

AF has been associated with AF in humans as well as in some murine models [57, 64]. However, the extent to which the structural substrate leads to the arrhythmia and the arrhythmias lead to changes in the substrate is unclear. Nakajima *et al.* developed a transgenic mouse model overexpressing mutant transforming growth factor-β1 (TGF-β1) in the heart [65]. Although equivalent levels of active TGF-β1 were present in the atria and the ventricles, the transgenic mice exhibited overt atrial but not ventricular fibrosis. These mice underwent surface electrocardiography and electrophysiological testing using an open-chest epicardial approach [66]. With aging, the transgenic mice exhibited lower-amplitude P waves. With burst atrial pacing and premature stimulation, four out of five transgenic and none of the wild-type mice were induced into AF. Each transgenic mouse was consistently inducible into AF with an average duration of 3 seconds per episode. This greater inducibility was not related to a change in the atrial effective refractory period. This model suggests a primary role of fibrosis in the pathogenesis of AF in mice.

RhoA overexpression mice

RhoA is a low-molecular-weight GTPase that is important for cardiac hypertrophy. Transgenic mice overexpressing either wild-type or a constitutively active form of RhoA using the α-myosin heavy chain promoter develop heart failure associated with atrial and ventricular dilatation [67]. EKG analysis during anesthesia with ketamine and pentobarbital demonstrated bradycardia not reversed by atropine, AV block and AF.

RTEF-1 overexpression mice

Cardiac myocytes respond to α1-adrenergic receptor stimulation by progressive hypertrophy accompanied by activation of fetal genes through signaling the binding sites of transcriptional enhancer factor-1 (TEF-1) family of transcriptor factors [68]. The overexpression of the TEF-1-related factor (RTEF-1) increases the α-adrenergic stimulation of skeletal muscles. Mice overexpressing cardiac-specific RTEF-1 were developed and studied at our institution. Compared with their wild-type counterparts the RTEF-1 transgenic mice develop progressive atrioventricular conduction disease, diastolic dysfunction, atrial dilatation and atrial arrhythmias [69]. With *in vivo* electrophysiological testing via a closed-chest approach, the transgenic mice exhibit longer PR and AH, but not HV intervals compared with the control mice, indicating delays in atrioventricular nodal conduction. During *in vitro* testing with optical mapping, mice over-expressing RTEF-1 exhibit slowing of both atrial and ventricular conduction velocities. During 56 hours of ambulatory monitoring, six out of six RTEF-1 transgenic and none of six control mice demonstrated self-terminating episodes of AF. These episodes were found to be enhanced by β-adrenergic stimulation with isoproterenol and suppressed by β-blockers.

Conclusions

The genetic and molecular basis of AF remains for the most part unknown. Transgenic mouse models have become essential tools for the determination of the pathophysiologic mechanisms of many cardiovascular diseases. While transgenic mouse models of AF have shed some light on these mechanisms, the technique remains relatively underused and a great deal remains to be learned. Gene products should be overexpressed in or conditionally deleted from the atrium using atrial promoters. Genes that modify AF can be identified by crossing transgenic and gene-targeted mice to mice already susceptible to AF. When genes causing the familial forms of AF are identified, mice harboring these mutations can be engineered. Ultimately, transgenic models of AF may help to unmask the major pathways involved in the genesis of this condition and may lead to new preventive and therapeutic modalities, possibly in the form of gene therapy.

References

1 Gordon JW. Transgenic animals. *Int Rev Cytol* 1989; **115**: 171–230.
2 Palmiter RD, Brinster RL. Germ-line transformation of mice. *Annu Rev Genet* 1986; **20**: 465–99.
3 Melton DW. Gene targeting in the mouse. *Bioessays* 1994; **16**: 633–8.
4 Van der Weyden L, Adams DJ, Bradley A. Tools for targeted manipulation of the mouse genome. *Physiol Genomics* 2002; **11**: 133–64.
5 Christensen G, Wang Y, Chien KR. Physiological assessment of complex cardiac pheno-types in genetically engineered mice. *Am J Physiol* 1997; **41**: H2513–14.
6 James JF, Hewett TE, Robbins J. Cardiac physiology in transgenic mice. *Circ Res* 1998; **82**: 407–15.
7 Priori SG, Barhanin J, Hauer NWR *et al.* Genetic and molecular basis of cardiac arrhyth-mias: impact on clinical management (Parts I and II). *Circulation* 1999; **99**: 518–28.
8 Priori SG, Barhanin J, Hauer NWR *et al.* Genetic and molecular basis of cardiac arrhyth-mias: Impact on clinical management (Parts III). *Circulation* 1999; **99**: 674–81.
9 Feinberg WM, Blackshear JL, Laupacis A, Kronmal R, Hart RG. Prevalence, age distribu-tion, and gender of patients with atrial fibrillation. *Arch Intern Med* 1995; **155**: 469–73.
10 Albers GW. Atrial fibrillation and stroke: three new studies, three remaining questions. *Arch Intern Med* 1994; **154**: 1443–8.
11 Wolff L. Familial auricular fibrillation. *N Engl J Med* 1943; **229**: 396–7.
12 Tikanoja T, Kirkinen P, Nikolajev K, Eresmaa L, Haring P. Familial atrial fibrillation with fetal onset. *Heart* 1998; **79**: 195–7.

13 Poret P, Mabo P, Deplace C *et al.* Isolated atrial fibrillation genetically-determined? Apropos of a familial history. *Arch Mal Coeur Vaiss* 1996; **89**: 1197–203.

14 Brugada R, Bashinski LL, Hill R, Roberts R. Familial atrial fibrillation is a genetically heterogeneous disease [abstract]. *J Am Coll Cardiol* 1998; **31**: 349A.

15 Ellinor PT, Shin JT, Moore RK, Yourger DM, MacRae CA. Locus for atrial fibrillation maps to chromosome 6q14–16. *Circulation* 2003; **107**: 2880–3.

16 Chen YH, Xu SJ, Bendahhou S *et al.* KCNQ1 gain-of-function mutation in familial atrial fibrillation. *Science* 2003; **299**: 251–4.

17 Lai LP, Su MJ, Yeh HM *et al.* Association of the human minK gene 38G allele with atrial fibrillation: evidence of possible genetic control on the pathogenesis of atrial fibrillation. *Am Heart J* 2002; **144**: 485–90.

18 Brudel BJ, Van Gelder IC, Henning RH *et al.* Ion channel remodeling is related to intraoperative atrial effective refractory periods in patients with paroxysmal and persistent atrial fibrillation. *Circulation* 2001; **103**: 684–90.

19 London B. Use of transgenic and gene-targeted mice to study K$^+$ channel function in the cardiovascular system. In: Archer SA, Rusch JF, eds. *Potassium Channels in Cardiovascular Biology.* New York: Plenum Publishing, 2001: 177–91.

20 Izumo S, Shioi T. Cardiac transgenic and gene-targeted mice as models of cardiac hypertrophy and failure: a problem of (new) riches. *J Card Failure* 1998; **4**: 349–61.

21 Neumann J, Boknik P, DePaoli-Roach AA *et al.* Targeted overexpression of phospholamban to mouse atrium depresses Ca^{2+} transport and contractility. *J Mol Cell Cardiol* 1998; **30**: 1991–2002.

22 Huang WY, Aramburu J, Douglas PS, Izumo S. Transgenic expression of green fluorescence protein can cause dilated cardiomyopathy. *Nat Med* 2000; **6**: 482–3.

23 Fishman GI. Timing is everything in life: conditional transgene expression in the cardiovascular system. *Circ Res* 1998; **82**: 837–44.

24 Huang JL, Morgan DJ. Influence of the pH on the uptake and pharmacokinetics of quinidine in the isolated perfused rat heart. *Pharmacol Toxicol* 1993; **73**: 115–19.

25 Nielsen CB, Mellemkjaer S, Nielsen-Kudsk F. Pinacidil uptake and effects in the isolated rabbit heart. *Pharmacol Toxicol* 1989; **25**: 30–4.

26 Pinney SP, Koller BS, Franz MR *et al.* Terfenadine increases the QT interval in isolated guinea pig heart. *J Cardiovasc Pharmcol* 1995; **64**: 14–19.

27 Stark G, Dhein S, Bachernegg M *et al.* Frequency-dependent effects of propafenone decrease with duration of ventricular tachycardia in isolated guinea pig hearts. *Eur J Pharmacol* 1994; **252**: 283–9.

28 London B, Baker LC, Lee JS *et al.* Calcium-dependent arrhythmias in transgenic mice with heart failure. *Am J Physiol Heart Circ Physiol* 2003; **284**: H431–41.

29 Baker LC, London B, Choi BR, Koren G, Salama G. Enhanced dispersion of repolarization and refractoriness in transgenic mouse hearts promotes reentrant ventricular tachycardia. *Circ Res* 2000; **86**: 396–407.

30 London B, Guo W, Pan X-H *et al.* Targeted replacement of KV1.5 in the mouse leads to loss of the 4-aminopyridine-sensitive component of I(K,slow) and resistance to drug-induced qt prolongation. *Circ Res* 2001; **88**: 940–6.

31 Saba S, Shusterman V, Usiene I, London B. Cardiac autonomic modulation by estrogen in female mice undergoing ambulatory monitoring and *in vivo* electrophysiologic testing. *Ann Non-Inv Electrocardiol* 2004; **9**:1420–8.

32 Shusterman V, Usiene I, Harrigal C *et al.* Strain-specific patterns of autonomic nervous system activity and heart failure susceptibility in mice. *Am J Physiol Heart Circ Physiol* 2002; **282**: H2076–83.

33 Varro A, Nakaya Y, Elharrar V *et al.* Effect of antiarrhythmic drugs on the cycle length-dependent action potential duration in dog purkinje and ventricular muscle fibers. *J Cardiovasc Pharmacol* 1986; **8**: 178–85.

34 Wang Z, Pelletier LC, Talajic M *et al.* Effects of flecainide and quinidine on human atrial action potentials: role of rate-dependence and comparison with guinea pig, rabbit, and dog tissues. *Circulation* 1990; **82**: 274–83.

35 Berul CI, Aronovitz MJ, Wang PJ *et al.* In vivo cardiac electrophysiologic studies in the mouse. *Circulation* 1996; **94**: 2641–8.

36 Saba S, VanderBrink BA, Luciano B *et al.* Localization of the site of conduction abnormality in a mouse model of myotonic dystrophy. *J Cardiovasc Electrophysiol* 1999; **10**: 1214–20.

37 Saba S, Wang PJ, Estes NAM III. Invasive cardiac electrophysiology in the mouse: techniques and applications. *Trends Cardiovasc Med* 2000; **10**: 122–32.

38 Goldberger AL, Pavelec RS. Vagally-mediated atrial fibrillation in dogs: conversion with bretylium tosylate. *Int J Cardiol* 1986; **13**: 47–55.

39 Wijffels MC, Kirchhof CJ, Dorland R, Allessie MA. Atrial fibrillation begets atrial fibrillation. A study in awake chronically instrumented goats. *Circulation* 1995; **92**: 1954–68.

40 Anadon MJ, Almendral J, Gonzalez P *et al.* Alcohol concentration determines the type of atrial arrhythmia induced in a porcine model of acute alcoholic intoxication. *PACE* 1996; **19**: 1962–7.

41 Friedrichs GS. Experimental models of atrial fibrillation/flutter. *J Pharmacol Toxicol Methods* 2000; **43**: 117–23.

42 Wakimoto H, Maguire CT, Kovoor P *et al.* Induction of atrial tachycardia and fibrillation in the mouse heart. *Cardiovasc Res* 2001; **50**: 463–73.

43 Schrickel JW, Bielik H, Yang A *et al.* Induction of atrial fibrillation in mice by rapid transesophageal atrial pacing. *Basic Res Cardiol* 2002; **97**: 452–60.

44 Wang YX, Zheng WM, Tan YH, Sheng BH. Effects of cycloprotobuxine-A on atrial fibrillation. *Zhongguo Yao Li Bao*1997; **18**: 245–50.

45 Wang YX, Zheng WM, Tan YH, Sheng BH. Anti atrial fibrillation effects of cycloprotobuxine-D and its electrophysiological mechanism studied on guinea pig atria. *Yao Xue Xue Bao* 1996; **31**: 481–6.

46 Miquerol L, Dupays L, Theveniau-Ruissy M *et al.* Gap junctional connexins in the developing mouse cardiac conduction system. *Novartis Found Symp* 2003; **250**: 80–98.

47 Gutstein DE, Morley GE, Tamaddon H *et al.* Conduction slowing and sudden arrhythmic death in mice with cardiac-restricted inactivation of connexin43. *Circ Res* 2001; **88**: 333–9.

48 Kumai M, Nishii K, Nkamura K, Takeda N, Suzuki M, Shibata Y. Loss of connexin45 causes a cushion defect in early cardiogenesis. *Development* 2000; **127**: 3501–12.

49 Kruger O, Plum A, Kim JS *et al.* Defective vascular development in connexin45-deficient mice. *Development* 2000; **127**: 4179–93.

50 Hagendorff A, Schumacher B, Kirchhoff S, Luderitz B, Willecke K. Conduction disturbances and increased atrial vulnerability in connexin40-deficient mice analyzed by transesophageal stimulation. *Circulation* 1999; **99**: 1508–15.

51 Verheule S, Van Batenburg CA, Coenjaerts FE *et al.* Cardiac conduction abnormalities in mice lacking the gap junction protein connexin40. *J Cardiovasc Electrophysiol* 1999; **10**: 1380–9.

52 VanderBrink BA, Salito C, Saba S *et al.* Insights into atrioventricular nodal and infrahisian conduction patterns using connexin-40 deficient mice. *J Cardiovasc Electrophysiol* 2000; **11**: 1270–6.

53 van der Velden HM, Ausma J, Rook MB *et al.* Gap junctional remodeling in relation to stabilization of atrial fibrillation in the goat. *Cardiovasc Res* 2000; **46**: 476–86.

54 Bettoni M, Zimmermann M. Autonomic tone variations before the onset of paroxysmal atrial fibrillation. *Circulation* 2002; **105**: 2753–9.

55 Kurachi Y, Tung R, Ito H, Nakajima T. G protein activation of cardiac muscarinic K⁺ channels. *Prog Neurobiol* 1992; **39**: 226–46.

56 Kovoor P, Wickman K, Maguire CT *et al.* Evaluation of the role of I_{KACh} in atrial fibrillation using a mouse knockout model. *J Am Coll Cardiol* 2001; **37**: 2136–43.

57 Hong CS, Cho MC, Kwak YG *et al.* Cardiac remodeling and atrial fibrillation in transgenic mice overexpressing junctin. *FASEB J* 2002; **16**: 1310–12.

58 Kirchhefer U, Neumann J, Bers DM *et al.* Impaired relaxation in transgenic mice overexpressing junctin. *Cardiovasc Res* 2003; **59**: 369–79.

59 Koh JT, Choi HH, Ahn KY *et al.* Cardiac characteristics of transgenic mice overexpressing Refsum disease gene-associated protein within the heart. *Biochem Biophys Res Commun* 2001; **286**: 1107–16.

60 Seedorf U, Raabe M, Ellinghaus P *et al.* Defective peroxisomal catabolism of branched fatty acyl coenzyme A in mice lacking the sterol carrier protein-2/sterol carrier protein-x gene function. *Genes Dev* 1998; **12**: 1189–201.

61 Middlekauff HR, Stevenson WG, Stevenson LW. Prognostic significance of atrial fibrillation in advanced heart failure. A study of 390 patients. *Circulation* 1999; **84**: 40–8.

62 Kubota T, McTiernan CF, Frye CS *et al.* Dilated cardiomyopathy in transgenic mice with cardiac-specific overexpression of tumor necrosis factor-alpha. *Circ Res* 1997; **81**: 627–35.

63 Kadokami T, McTiernan CF, Kubota T, Frye CS, Feldman AM. Sex-related survival differences in murine cardiomyopathy are associated with differences in TNF-receptor expression. *J Clin Invest* 2000; **106**: 589–97.

64 Frustaci A, Chimenti C, Bellocci F *et al.* Histological substrate of atrial biopsies in patients with lone atrial fibrillation. *Circulation* 1997; **96**: 1180–4.

65 Nakajima H, Nakajima HO, Salcher O *et al.* Atrial but not ventricular fibrosis in mice expressing a mutant transforming growth factor-beta (1) transgene in the heart. *Circ Res* 2000; **86**: 571–9.

66 Raiesdana A, Verheule S, Nakajima H, Nakajima H, Field L, Olgin JE. Inducibility of atrial arrhythmias in transgenic mice with selective atrial fibrosis due to overexpression of TGF-β1 [abstract]. *PACE* 2001; **24**: 549.

67 Sah VP, Minamisawa S, Tam SP *et al.* Cardiac-specific overexpression of RhoA results in sinus and atrioventricular nodal dysfunction and contractile failure. *J Clin Invest* 1999; **103**: 1627–34.

68 Stewart AF, Suzow J, Kubota T, Ueyama T, Chen HH. Transcription factor RTEF-1 mediates alpha1-adrenergic reactivation of the fetal gene program in cardiac myocytes. *Circ Res* 1998; **83**: 43–9.

69 Stewart AFRS, Maeda T, Ueyama T, Zhu C, Koretsky AP, London B. Conduction defects progressing to atrial fibrillation and altered channel expression in RTEF-1 transgenic mice [abstract]. *Circulation* 2000; **102**: II–153.

CHAPTER 5

Atrial Plasticity

Prashanthan Sanders, Joseph B. Morton, Paul B. Sparks, Jonathan M. Kalman

The clinical observation that paroxysmal atrial fibrillation (AF) becomes increasingly frequent and eventually persistent has resulted in animal and human studies to determine the possible substrate that creates and then maintains AF. A number of studies have demonstrated that the atrial substrate has the property of plasticity; that is, adaptation (remodeling) to a varying physiological milieu. In this chapter, we will review aspects of electrical, structural and mechanical remodeling.

Electrical remodeling

Wijffels *et al.* described the concept of atrial electrical remodeling due to AF in a landmark study in conscious chronically instrumented goats, providing the seminal observation that 'AF begets AF' [1]. These investigators observed that, while induced AF was initially short-lived, the artificial maintenance of AF resulted in a progressive increase in the duration of AF to become sustained with time. This persistence of AF was associated with shortening of the fibrillatory interval and the atrial effective refractory period (ERP) and a propensity to develop AF with single extrastimuli. Other animal studies have observed remarkably similar and consistent changes in atrial ERP associated with rapid atrial rates or AF [2–5]. Similar studies in humans have observed that even brief durations of AF resulted in a reduction of atrial ERP. Daoud *et al.* demonstrated that just a few minutes of induced AF in humans was sufficient to cause significant fall in atrial ERP [6].

A number of clinical studies have studied the effects of chronic atrial arrhythmias on atrial electrophysiology. Kumagai *et al.* studied patients with lone AF of greater than 1 year's duration and observed that following cardioversion to sinus rhythm there was a significantly abbreviated atrial ERP, prolongation of the P wave duration, increased intra-atrial conduction time, and fragmented atrial activity [7]. Others have also provided evidence to suggest that there is an increase in the heterogeneity of atrial ERP as a result of chronic AF in humans [8]. Franz *et al.* found significantly shorter monophasic action potential duration in the right atrium following cardioversion of AF or flutter compared with a control group [9]. Sparks *et al.* demonstrated that, following the termination of chronic atrial flutter by radiofrequency ablation, atrial ERPs at the lateral right atrium, septum and coronary sinus were significantly shorter 15 and 30 minutes after termination of atrial flutter compared with 3 weeks later [10]. In addition to the changes in atrial ERP as a result of chronic atrial arrhythmias, Yu *et al.* also observed depressed atrial conduction time along the lateral right atrium and coronary sinus following the cardioversion of chronic AF compared with controls [11]. These authors also performed daily studies for 4 days following cardioversion and found no improvement in atrial conduction but significant improvement in the atrial ERP.

Several groups have also demonstrated the occurrence of sinus node remodeling as a result of atrial arrhythmia. Elvan *et al.* demonstrated significant prolongation of sinus node recovery time, corrected sinus node recovery time, and the intrinsic sinus cycle length with 2–6 weeks of AF in a canine model [12]. Sinus node remodeling has also been observed in humans. Following the cardioversion of chronic lone AF, the sinus node recovery time was significantly longer than in control patients [13, 14]. Manios *et al.* also observed that reversal of sinus node remodeling due to AF does not occur within 24 hours after cardioversion and may be associated with a trend to recurrence of AF, raising the possibility that sinus node dysfunction forms part of the rate-related remodeling milieu that predisposes to recurrent AF [14]. This phenomenon of sinus node remodeling again does not appear unique to AF but has also been demonstrated following the termination of chronic atrial flutter [15]. Irrespective of the mechanism by which sinus node remodeling occurs due to rapid atrial rates, an increase in the time window due to sinus bradycardia can strongly facilitate the conditions for AF occurrence by increasing atrial ectopy and the dispersion of ERP [16]. A fall in ERP, loss of rate adaptation, increased heterogeneity of ERP, regional conduction slowing and sinus node dysfunction have all been demonstrated as a result of rapid atrial rates or AF. All of these electrophysiological perturbations are favorable to the maintenance of further AF either by shortening the wavelength or increasing the heterogeneity of the electrophysiological characteristics of the atria.

Several cellular changes documented to occur in association with rapid atrial rates have been evaluated as possible mechanisms for the observed electrophysiological changes. At least acutely, if not in the long term, cellular calcium overload is apparent [17, 18]. Yue *et al.* in a canine model of AF demonstrated a decrease of calcium-independent transient outward current (I_{to}) and the L-type calcium current ($I_{Ca,L}$) density with tachycardia [19]. Similar findings have also been observed in humans with AF [20–37]. Furthermore, inhibition of the $I_{Ca,L}$ of an isolated cell by nifedipine mimics the changes in action potential seen with tachycardia, while an agonist of the receptor (Bay K 8644) reverses these abnormalities, suggesting that suppression of this receptor may have a critical role in the observed changes in refractoriness [19]. Tieleman *et al.* have also demonstrated significant attenuation of the changes in ERP associated with 24 hours of rapid atrial rates following the administration of verapamil in an animal model [24]. Daoud *et al.* have also observed similar attenuation of the changes in ERP in a clinical study of brief duration AF by the pre-administration of verapamil [6]. However, it seems that remodeling induced by longer durations of atrial arrhythmia is not reduced by diltiazem [25] or verapamil [26], but is substantially attenuated by mibefradil (a selective T-type calcium blocker), suggesting a role for the T-type calcium channel in the remodeling associated with longer durations of atrial arrhythmia [27]. However, another study found that the T-type calcium channel and the calcium-dependent chloride channel densities were unaffected by tachycardia [19]. In addition, changes in sodium ion channels have been observed. Gaspo *et al.* observed downregulation of the rapid sodium current (I_{Na}), a phenomenon that occurred over a longer time-frame than changes seen in calcium channels [28]. These alterations in I_{Na} correlate with changes in atrial conduction velocity observed with maintained atrial tachycardia, and as such may contribute to the slowing of conduction velocity associated with AF. A variety of potassium channels have been studied following rapid atrial pacing in dogs. Van Wagoner *et al.* reported a decrease in I_{to} and I_{sus} (along with Kv1.5 subunit protein) in patients with AF [29]. Bosch *et al.* observed a decreased I_{to} and an increase in both I_{K1} and I_{KACh} densities in right atrial myocytes of patients with AF [20]. Brundel *et al.* studied the protein levels of Kv4.3, Kv1.5, HERG, minK and Kir3.1 in patients with AF and found that they were reduced compared with controls [22]. However, the functional significance of these changes for atrial electrophysiology and arrhythmia promotion is unknown.

While rapidly occurring changes in atrial electrophysiology have been demonstrated even with atrial arrhythmias of brief duration [38], the development of persistent atrial arrhythmias in humans is a long-term process. Although atrial electrical remodeling associated with atrial arrhythmias was initially considered to result in the cascade of cause and effect that led paroxysmal AF to become persistent and then chronic, not all studies have supported this hypothesis. Garratt *et al.* studied the effect of recurrent episodes of paroxysmal AF in the goat model [39] and found that even after three such episodes of AF of 5 days' duration, each separated by 2 days of sinus rhythm, there was no additive atrial remodeling. Furthermore, if the cascade of cause and effect is central to the progression of paroxysmal AF to chronic AF, then not only should AF beget AF by atrial remodeling but sinus rhythm should also beget sinus rhythm. To evaluate this concept, Fynn *et al.* studied the clinical benefit of early repeated cardioversion of AF to sinus rhythm and found that even with an aggressive policy of immediate restoration of sinus rhythm each time AF occurred, there was no decrease in the episodes of AF [40]. While repeated early cardioversion did not prevent the development of AF in these patients, other studies have observed that even when sinus rhythm is maintained the substrate for AF remains present. Rodriguez *et al.* report that in patients implanted with an atrial defibrillator for a 14-month period AF was still inducible with single extrastimuli at least 1000 hours after the last AF episode [41]. Furthermore, Ramanna *et al.* observed that patients with idiopathic AF showed increased dispersion of ERP and increased AF inducibility even distant from a clinical paroxysm of AF [42]. These authors suggested that these findings may reflect the presence of a primary substrate for AF.

These studies hint at the importance of factors which may create the primary underlying substrate for AF, producing the milieu both for the initial development of paroxysmal AF and also for the progression to chronic AF.

The heterogeneity in mechanisms underlying AF is reflected by the diversity of pathophysiological processes that create the substrate for this arrhythmia. While recent studies have emphasized the importance of atrial remodeling due to rapid atrial rates, much attention has also been directed to the role of stretch (mechano-electric feedback) in the atria. Atrial stretch plays an apparent role in the development of AF in a wide spectrum of clinical conditions, ranging from the acute effects of supraventricular tachycardias and myocardial infarction to chronic conditions such as heart failure, mitral valve disease, atrial septal defects and asynchronous ventricular (VVI) pacing.

Animal studies of the impact of acute atrial stretch on atrial electrophysiology have yielded divergent results. Kaseda and Zipes demonstrated an increase in atrial ERP due to atrial stretch produced by simultaneous atrioventricular pacing both in anesthetized open-chest dogs and in chronically instrumented conscious dogs [43]. Increases in atrial ERP were observed in the right and left atria and at the interatrial septum, and persisted despite autonomic blockade. Subsequently, Satoh and Zipes demonstrated this increase in atrial ERP to be heterogeneous [44]. In this model anesthetized open-chest dogs had stretch induced by fluid loading and simultaneous atrioventricular pacing. Under these conditions of increased ERP heterogeneity, AF inducibility also increased. Wijffels *et al.* also used acute fluid loading to produce atrial stretch [45]. The sudden volume load of 0.5 to 1 litre of Hemaccel produced significant increases in the atrial size and atrial pressure, and increased left and right atrial ERP. Sideris *et al.* also demonstrated that acute volume overload in anesthetized dogs resulted in a significant increase in right atrial ERP, interatrial conduction time and the susceptibility to AF induction by rapid atrial stimulation [46].

In contrast to these studies in the whole animal, isolated heart preparations have demonstrated an abbreviation of atrial ERP. In Langendorff-perfused rabbit hearts, Ravelli *et al.* observed a decrease in left and right atrial ERP associated with acute atrial dilatation [47]. Atrial pressure increases in this model were performed by ligation of the pulmonary and caval veins and varying the exit of perfusion fluid from the pulmonary artery. At low pressures (less than 7–8 cm H_2O) no changes in atrial ERP were observed. These findings are similar to those of an isolated Langendorff-perfused guinea-pig heart study, in which stretch was induced by inflation of an intra-atrial balloon catheter [48]. In this study the left atrial monophasic action potential (MAP) was studied, showing a decrease in the MAP duration (50%) due to a decrease in the duration of the plateau phase but a paradoxical increase in the MAP duration (90%) due to the presence of early afterdepolarizations. These afterdepolarizations produced atrial premature beats and were associated with an increase in atrial arrhythmias.

Studies in humans of the effects of acute atrial stretch have also yielded quite variable effects on atrial ERP. Calkins *et al.* reported that simultaneous atrioventricular pacing produced no change in atrial ERP at a drive cycle length of 400 ms in patients without structural heart disease, and they observed no increase in the frequency of AF induction [49]. However, the same group found that atrial ERP shortened in response to acute changes in atrial pressure brought about by pacing just the final two beats of the drive train at an atrioventricular interval of 0 ms [50]. Tse *et al.* also used acute simultaneous atrioventricular pacing to cause atrial stretch and again observed a decrease in right atrial ERP accompanied by increased inducibility of AF [51]. In contrast, Klein *et al.* found an increase in atrial ERP associated with an increase in atrial pressure occurring when the atrioventricular interval was decreased from 160 to 0 ms [52]. Similarly Chen *et al.* found a non-uniform increase in atrial ERP associated with an increase in atrial pressure during simultaneous atrioventricular pacing in patients without structural heart disease [53]. There was a significant increase in the atrial ERP measured at the distal coronary sinus and the posterior lateral right atrium but not at the right atrial appendage. As a result they also observed an increase in the dispersion of ERP [53]. Several studies have also evaluated the impact of atrial stretch during supraventricular tachycardia, when near simultaneous activation of the ventricle and atria occurs. Klein *et al.* observed an increase in right atrial ERP associated with an increase in right atrial pressure [52]. Similarly, Chen *et al.* observed an increase in atrial ERP and dispersion of ERP with an increase in atrial pressure with supraventricular tachycardia [54].

The reason why studies on acute atrial stretch have produced such varying observations is not readily apparent but may relate in part to methodology and to the number of sites sampled. As some of the above studies have suggested, more important than the absolute change in ERP at a single site may be the relative changes in ERP between regions that lead to increased heterogeneity of ERP.

In contrast to the array of results produced by contraction–excitation feedback seen in acute atrial stretch, studies of chronic atrial stretch have yielded more consistent results. Boyden and Hoffman evaluated the effects of chronic right atrial stretch on atrial electrophysiology [55]. In a canine model, excising the septal cusp of the tricuspid valve through a right atriotomy created tricuspid incompetence, and together with constricting the pulmonary artery resulted in right atrial enlargement. At 2 weeks and for 20–30 weeks after surgery these dogs were more susceptible to atrial arrhythmias by extrastimuli than sham-operated dogs. Ultrastructural studies on these dogs demonstrated hypertrophy of fibres and some increase in the connective tissue between cells. However, there was no change in the right atrial muscle fibre membrane potential. In a separate study by Boyden *et al.*, 23 dogs with spontaneous mitral valve fibrosis and left atrial enlargement were studied [56]. Of these dogs, 13 had intermittent atrial arrhythmias and 10 had chronic AF. There was no difference in the action potential duration between these two groups. Structural studies in the left atrium of these dogs demonstrated a reduced number of muscle cell layers and an unusually large amount of connective tissue between greatly hypertrophied cells. These authors concluded that the altered susceptibility to arrhythmia might not require significant abnormalities of cellular electrophysiology. Boyden *et al.* further extended their original observations by studying the characteristics of the atria in spontaneously occurring feline cardiomyopathy [66]. These investigators observed non-excitability of some atrial cells and again demonstrated the presence of marked structural abnormalities, including large amounts of interstitial fibrosis, cellular hypertrophy and degeneration, and thickened basement membranes [57]. Li *et al.* evaluated the effects of chronic atrial stretch due to ventricular pacing-induced congestive heart failure in a canine model [58]. In these animals, 5 weeks of rapid ventricular pacing induced significant clinical congestive heart failure with increases in left and right atrial pressures. This was associated with atrial structural changes different than those associated with AF: there was no change in the atrial ERP at longer cycle lengths but a significant increase in ERP at shorter cycle lengths and no change in the heterogeneity of ERP. While there was no change in the conduction velocity they observed a significant increase in the heterogeneity of conduction due to marked structural abnormalities with interstitial fibrosis. Presumably as a result of these abnormalities in conduction and atrial structure, and despite the increase in atrial ERP, these animals demonstrated a significant increase in the duration of AF. Using the same model, these investigators observed that this substrate for AF may also be modified by other factors, such as autonomic tone [59] and the use of angiotensin-converting enzyme inhibitors [60].

Verheule *et al.* studied the electrophysiological consequences of chronic atrial stretch produced by 1 month of mitral regurgitation in a canine model [61]. Mitral regurgitation was produced by avulsion of the mitral valve. These investigators demonstrated a uniform increase in atrial ERP and no significant change in atrial conduction velocity. There was, however, a significant increase in the inducibility of sustained AF, which was not based on a decrease in wavelength. Pathological evaluation of the atria from these animals showed areas of increased interstitial fibrosis and chronic inflammation, and this structural change may be the critical factor in the increased propensity to sustained AF in this model. It was suggested that regional fibrosis may potentially be associated with preferential regional abnormalities in conduction [61].

Studies on the effects of chronic atrial stretch feedback in humans are much more limited. Chen *et al.* studied ten patients with atrial dilatation and no history of atrial arrhythmias, and found significantly longer atrial ERP compared with 20 control patients with normal atrial size [62]. Sparks *et al.* evaluated the effects of long-term asynchronous ventricular pacing on the electrical properties and mechanical function of the atria [63]. This study was a prospective randomized comparison between 18 patients paced in VVI mode and 12 patients paced in DDD mode for 3 months. After chronic VVI pacing, atrial ERP increased significantly in a non-uniform fashion at all sites evaluated (the lateral right atrium, right atrial appendage, right atrial septum and distal coronary sinus). This was also associated with prolongation of the P wave duration and sinus node remodeling [63]. In a parallel study, these authors also demonstrated significant enlargement of the atria associated with impairment of atrial mechanical function, as evidenced by a decrease in the left atrial appendage emptying velocities and fractional area change [64]. Importantly, these studies also documented that these changes associated with 3 months of VVI pacing could be reversed by 3 months of physiological (DDD) pacing.

Structural remodeling

More recently, Willems *et al.* have postulated the role of a 'second factor', identified as the structural changes that result from atrial arrhythmia, in the maintenance of AF [65]. Ausma and co-workers have studied the effect of AF on atrial structural remodeling in studies of chronically instrumented goats. While atrial electrical remodeling was found to occur at the onset of AF and appeared to be completed after 2 weeks, the first obvious signs of structural remodeling became apparent after 2–4 weeks of AF and reached a steady state between 8 and 16 weeks [31, 32]. These investigators have described the structural abnormalities in their model of AF as representing dedifferentiation of atrial myocytes representing adaptive changes due to arrhythmia [33]. Pathological studies in humans have also identified degenerative changes and fibrosis within the atria of patients with atrial arrhythmias [34–41, 66–73]. While animal studies have not identified morphological changes associated with apoptosis [32], such changes were observed in a human pathology study of patients with AF [35].

Ausma *et al.* have recently reported that reverse remodeling of these structural abnormalities occurs at a much slower rate than the tachycardia-associated changes in atrial ERP [32]. In a canine model of AF in association with mitral regurgitation, Everett *et al.* did not observe any reverse remodeling of the structural changes 2 weeks after cardioversion of AF [66].

Integral to the structural remodelling process is the development of abnormalities in cell-to-cell connections. Although clinical and experimental studies of AF have demonstrated significant remodeling of the gap junction proteins of connexin40 and 43, there are conflicting data regarding these changes in experimental models. Elvan *et al.* showed upregulation of connexin43 expression in dogs with atrial tachycardia maintained for 10–14 weeks by electrical stimulation [67]. However, in a similar goat model connexin43 mRNA and protein remained unchanged and an altered distribution of connexin40 was observed [68]. In contrast, in humans with AF, Kostin *et al.* demonstrated a reduced level of connexin43, suggesting perhaps that there is interspecies variation in this protein [36]. Kostin *et al.* have also demonstrated displacement of N-cadherin and desmoplakin from the cell termini to the lateral borders in humans with chronic atrial fibrillation [36].

Other factors have also been demonstrated in the extracellular matrix in association with atrial arrhythmia. Rocken *et al.* found increased isolated atrial amyloidosis associated with AF in patients having cardiac surgery [69]. Arndt *et al.* have demonstrated that in patients with AF there is increased expression of ADAMs (*a d*isintegrin *a*nd *m*etalloproteinase), a large family of membrane-bound glycoproteins that are known to regulate cell–cell and cell–matrix inter-actions and may thereby influence the architecture of cardiac tissue [70].

Emerging evidence indicates a role for angiotensin, a potent stimulus for the development of fibrosis, in the development of atrial structural remodeling in response to atrial arrhythmia. Nakashima *et al.* demonstrated that treatment with an angiotensin-converting enzyme inhibitor (captopril) or angiotensin-II receptor antagonist (candesartan) abolished atrial electrical remodeling in a canine model of rapid atrial pacing for 180 minutes [71]. Willems *et al.* observed that, together with atrial electrical remodeling, there is a significant and rapid increase in angiotensin-II levels associated with rapid atrial rates [65]. Goette *et al.* demonstrated that the atrial expression of angiotensin-converting enzyme is increased in patients with AF, possibly leading to angiotensin II-dependent progressive atrial fibrosis [72]. These observations have been extended by the same group to demonstrate changes in angiotensin-II receptor types in patients with AF, with downregulation of the atrial AT_1 receptor and upregulation of the atrial AT_2 receptor proteins compared with controls [73].

Mechanical remodeling

The most devastating complication associated with AF is that of cardioembolic stroke. The risk of stroke in patients with AF increases from 1.5% per year between the ages of 50 and 59 years to 24% per year in patients over the age of 80 years [74]. In patients with AF, in the absence of rheumatic heart disease the risk of stroke is five-fold greater after adjusting for other stroke risk factors [75], while in patients with rheumatic heart disease there is a 17.5-fold increased risk [76]. There is also an increased incidence of silent cerebral infarction [77]. Furthermore, evidence suggests that strokes complicating AF have increased severity of neurological deficit and are twice as likely to be fatal [78].

Atrial mechanical dysfunction or mechanical remodeling that develops in response to atrial arrhythmias and the transient period of atrial mechanical 'stunning' following cardioversion of AF have been implicated in the genesis of thromboembolic stroke [79–81]. Recent studies have made similar mechanistic observations in patients with atrial flutter [82–84]. Embolic events associated with cardioversion were initially thought to be a result of the expulsion of pre-formed atrial thrombus on resumption of sinus rhythm [85]. However, Black *et al.* found that the exclusion of thrombus by transesophageal echocardiography prior to cardioversion did not preclude embolic events after cardioversion, demonstrating the importance of the transient period of stunning after car-dioversion in the genesis of thromboembolic phenomena [86]. Consequently, current management guidelines stipulate anticoagulation for 3–4 weeks prior to and following cardioversion of AF of greater than 48 hours' duration or when the duration of AF is not known [87, 88]. While these guidelines are based on the presumption that significant atrial mechanical remodeling does not occur within the first 48 hours of AF, an understanding of the time course of atrial mechanical remodeling and its relationship to the rapidly developing electrical remodeling is still evolving.

In a canine model of rapid atrial pacing, Louie *et al.* demonstrated that 60 minutes of rapid atrial pacing resulted in a 64% reduction in mitral A wave velocity and a 49% reduction in the left atrial appendage emptying velocity (LAAEV) [89]. These observations in the canine model have been extended by Altemose *et al.*, who documented a progressive decline in left atrial fractional shortening and LAAEV over the first 5 hours of rapid atrial pacing, demonstrating a plateau effect at 180 minutes for left atrial fractional shortening and at 120 minutes for LAAEV [90]. Schotten *et al.*, in a goat model of AF of 5 hours duration, confirmed the rapid onset of atrial mechanical remodeling and demonstrated that, in the first days of AF, atrial electrical and mechanical remodeling go hand in hand [91]. Sanders *et al.* have studied the time course of atrial mechanical remodeling over a 6-week period of rapid atrial pacing in a conscious ovine model with the use of intracardiac echocardiography (unpublished data). This study demonstrated the rapid development of atrial mechanical remodeling with a decrease in the LAAEV that was rapid in the first 48 hours, reached a plateau at 2 weeks but was progressive over the 6 weeks. However, left atrial spontaneous echocardiographic contrast (LASEC) developed in only half the animals over a significantly longer period and no animal developed atrial thrombus. This study also indicated that atrial electrical and mechanical remodeling occurs over the same time interval.

Similar data in humans are limited because of the inability to study the time course of remodeling over a prolonged period. Daoud *et al.* studied the effects of 15.3 ± 3.8 minutes of induced AF in patients with no structural heart disease, and demonstrated significant decrease in LAAEV from 70 ± 20 to 63 ± 20 cm/s [92]. However, a similar study by Sparks *et al.* in patients with structural heart disease demonstrated that 15–20 minutes of AF was not associated with a post-reversion change in LAAEV, although 58% of patients developed new or increased LASEC during AF [93]. These data suggest that atrial mechanical remodeling develops rapidly, and while further clinical studies are awaited to evaluate the time course of atrial mechanical remodeling and the associated risk of stroke, it cannot necessarily be assumed that short durations of AF are not associated with a risk of thromboembolic complications.

Atrial mechanical stunning following the cardioversion of atrial arrhythmias was at least initially attributed to the direct current energy used for electrical cardioversion, with documentation of resultant cardiac injury by the release of cardiac muscle enzymes. However, atrial mechanical stunning has also been demonstrated with the use of low-energy endocardial cardioversion [94]. To evaluate the effect of the cardioversion itself on atrial mechanical function, Dodds *et al.* evaluated atrial mechanical function following the delivery of direct current endocardial or transthoracic shocks to patients in ventricular tachycardia, demonstrating no significant effect on atrial mechanical function [95]. Similarly, Sparks *et al.* delivered both graded endocardial and transthoracic shocks to patients in sinus rhythm and demonstrated no effect on atrial mechanical function [96]. These studies have conclusively shown that atrial mechanical dysfunction is not due to the direct current shock itself. The observations that atrial mechanical stunning also follows pharmacological cardioversion and occurs in patients with AF who revert spontaneously has led to the search for a common etiological mechanism [97, 98]. The development of atrial mechanical stunning on termination of atrial flutter is also recognized, following electrical cardioversion [99, 100], pharmacological cardioversion, pace termination [99, 100] and radiofrequency ablation [82, 83]. Together, these reports suggest that atrial mechanical stunning observed following reversion to sinus rhythm develops independently of the mode of cardioversion, and implicates the preceding tachyarrhythmia in the development of atrial mechanical stunning, a form of tachycardia-mediated atrial cardiomyopathy [4]. Atrial mechanical remodeling or dysfunction as a result of atrial arrhythmias could largely be attributed to the structural abnormalities that are known to result from atrial arrhythmia. However, while these processes take weeks to develop, atrial mechanical remodeling is observed with short durations of atrial arrhythmia, suggesting a role for more functional cellular mechanisms in the development of atrial mechanical dysfunction in response to atrial arrhythmia. Isolated cardiac muscle studies have demonstrated a positive force–frequency relationship or an inotropic effect of rate in ventricular myocardial fibres from normal hearts, while in failing ventricular myocardium this relationship is reversed [101]. The central regulator of cardiac contractility is calcium [102], frequency-dependent force generation being mediated through intracellular calcium balance [103–105]. Studies of the effects of atrial arrhythmias themselves in animal models have suggested a role for altered calcium handling [18] and intracellular calcium accumulation [17]. Using atrial tissue from AF patients, Schotten *et al.* demonstrated a concentration-dependent increase in the force of contraction during isoproterenol or calcium stimulation, relative to tissue from non-AF patients [23].

These observations have been extended to the whole atrium in a clinical study of patients with chronic atrial flutter undergoing cardioversion by radiofrequency ablation [106]. In this study, after the development of atrial mechanical stunning on termination of atrial flutter, atrial mechanical function, as determined by LAAEV and LASEC, was observed to be improved by pacing the atria at faster rates. Atrial mechanical function was also observed to normalize with the post-pacing pause. Together, these studies suggest a functional mechanism for atrial mechanical dysfunction associated with AF, and a critical role of cellular calcium handling. Schotten *et al.* have additionally demonstrated a decrease in the L-type calcium-current and an upregulation of the sodium–calcium exchanger without alteration of contractile proteins, suggesting that the extrusion of calcium from the cell by adaptive mechanisms that are activated by AF may result in relative cellular calcium depletion [23, 107]. This manifests clinically as atrial mechanical dysfunction.

While the above studies suggest that atrial mechanical dysfunction associated with AF is not caused by the disruption of the contractile apparatus itself, longer durations of AF are known to be associated with atrial structural remodeling that may be expected to result in impairment of atrial contractility [35, 108]. Sanders *et al.* have demonstrated divergent effects of pacing and isoproterenol in a clinical study of patients with AF of short and long duration (3.2 ± 0.5 months versus 57.7 ± 8.7 months), suggesting a possible role of structural abnormalities in atrial mechanical dysfunction [109]. In this study, while patients cardioverted from short-duration AF demonstrated significant improvement and reversal of atrial mechanical function with these maneuvers, patients cardioverted from prolonged AF demonstrated an attenuated response. Furthermore, there was a significantly attenuated response of atrial mechanical function with the post-pacing pause beat. These findings infer that the structural abnormalities resulting from prolonged duration of arrhythmia may additionally contribute to the atrial contractile dysfunction associated with AF.

Mondillo *et al.* studied various coagulation factors and indirect markers of endothelial dysfunction (D-dimer, tissue plasminogen activator, plasminogen activator inhibitor, von Willebrand factor and soluble thrombomodulin) [110]. They demonstrated a significant increase in and correlation between endothelial and coagulation factors in patients with lone AF, suggesting that endothelial dysfunction due to AF may lead to abnormalities in coagulation. Direct measures of the endothelial dysfunction during AF have demonstrated overexpression of mRNA and protein levels of endothelin-1 in atrial tissue during AF, suggesting a possible paracrine function in the remodeling process [111]. A recent thought-provoking study by Cai *et al.* using a rapid pacing model of AF in pigs observed that 1 week of rapid atrial pacing was associated with a significant decrease in endothelial nitric oxide synthetase and nitric oxide production and an increase in the expression of plasminogen activator inhibitor 1 in the left atrial myocardium [112]. As nitric oxide has an antithrombotic effect, they conclude that the decrease in nitric oxide synthetase may be the potential mechanism of thromboembolic complications associated with AF.

Synthesis: clinical substrates for atrial fibrillation

A range of clinical conditions are associated with AF; recent studies have examined the atrial remodeling in the following conditions.

Mitral regurgitation

Tieleman *et al.* have recently presented electrophysiological data on atrial ERP performed at the time of cardiac surgery in a heterogeneous group of patients: 15 with chronic AF, 16 with paroxysmal AF and 15 with no history of AF [113]. Of these patients, 22 had a history of mitral regurgitation. They report that mitral regurgitation was associated with prolongation of the atrial ERP irrespective of the underlying atrial rhythm, compared with the patients without mitral regurgitation. This observation is consistent with findings from animal models of mitral regurgitation described above and again suggests the substrate for AF in mitral regurgitation is likely to be independent of atrial ERP.

We have studied ten patients with severe mitral regurgitation due to mitral valve prolapse who had not previously developed AF (unpublished data). Patients with rheumatic valvular pathology were excluded. These patients demonstrated an increase in atrial ERP, significant prolongation of the P wave duration and regional conduction delays when compared with age-matched controls. We believe that these conduction heterogeneities may be responsible for increased propensity to AF.

Mitral stenosis

While much less frequent as a cause of AF in Western society, mitral stenosis due to rheumatic heart disease is frequently complicated by the development of AF and remains a significant illness in many countries worldwide. Fan *et al.* studied the electrophysiological findings in the right atrium in 31 patients with mitral valve stenosis at the time of percutaneous mitral commissurotomy [114]. Of these, 19 were in chronic AF and 12 in sinus rhythm at the time of the procedure. Following cardioversion of AF, these patients demonstrated significantly abbreviated atrial ERP, and sinus node remodeling, but no significant difference in atrial conduction delay to extrastimuli compared with patients in sinus rhythm. At a repeat study 3 months following mitral commissurotomy, the atrial ERP had increased significantly in patients cardioverted from AF. However, this study did not include a control group and the impact of atrial enlargement independent of AF was not addressed in detail. Furthermore, it might be expected that in patients with rheumatic heart disease the primary disease process would contribute to the substrate for AF.

Congestive heart failure

In developed countries congestive heart failure is the most common condition to be complicated by the development of AF, occurring in up to 30% of patients during the course of the disease. Sanders *et al.* studied 21 patients with congestive heart failure (left ventricular ejection fraction (LVEF) 25.2 ± 1.3%; 11 with idiopathic dilated and 10 with chronic ischemic cardiomyopathy) and 21 age-matched controls [115]. Patients with congestive heart failure demonstrated an increase in atrial ERP with no change in the heterogeneity of ERP. There was an increase in atrial conduction time, prolongation of the P wave duration and impairment of sinus node function. These patients also had evidence of anatomically determined conduction delay along the crista terminalis. Electroanatomical mapping confirmed significant regional conduction slowing but, importantly, also demonstrated regions of low atrial voltage and electrical silence (or scar). In accordance with the electrophysiological and electroanatomical abnormalities, these patients with congestive heart failure demonstrated an increased propensity for AF with single extra-stimuli and induced AF was more often sustained. Thus, in patients with congestive heart failure the substrate for AF may be predominantly due to the development of structural abnormalities and conduction delay rather than changes in atrial ERP, as occurs in remodeling due to rapid atrial rates. Indeed, pathological series in patients with cardiomyopathy have suggested the presence of significant atrial structural abnormalities [116].

Atrial septal defect

Morton *et al.* studied the right atrial electrophysiological properties of 13 patients with hemodynamically significant atrial septal defects and compared these with those of 17 age-matched controls [117]. These patients demonstrated an increase in atrial ERP at all right atrial sites evaluated, without a change in measured ERP heterogeneity. These patients also demonstrated significant prolongation of the P-wave duration, impairment of sinus node function and anatomically determined conduction delay at the crista terminalis. Again, the substrate for atrial arrhythmia development in this process was related to structural change and regional conduction abnormalities rather than to absolute refractory period. Interestingly, follow-up studies 6 months after closure of the atrial septal defect did not demonstrate significant reversal of these abnormalities despite reduction in atrial size.

Sinus node dysfunction

Sinus node function is often associated with AF [9]. While there may be numerous reasons for this, the detailed electrophysiological basis for this relationship remains poorly understood. Small series have observed prolonged P-wave duration and prolonged and fractionated atrial electrograms in patients with sinus node disease [118–121]. De Sisti *et al.* recently reported a retrospective review of patients with sinus node disease who had electrophysiological assessment and found no change in ERP at the high right atrium at a cycle length of 600 ms but a significant increase in electrogram duration both during the drive cycle length and extrastimuli, compared with controls [122]. However, their control group was not age-matched and consisted of patients with syncope or other conduction abnormalities. Sanders *et al.* studied 16 patients with symptomatic sick sinus syndrome diagnosed by unexplained sinus bradycardia (<40 beats/minute) or sinus pauses (>3.0 seconds) and 16 age-matched controls [123]. These patients were found to have prolonged P-wave duration, prolonged atrial conduction time, regional conduction delay, and prolongation of atrial ERP at each right atrial site evaluated. Electroanatomical mapping demonstrated the diffuse loss of atrial voltage, particularly prominent along the crista terminalis (region of the sinus pacemaker complex) with regions of electrical silence (scar). The residual sinus node complex became localized to a small region of the crista terminalis that was usually in the low posterior atrium and associated with the largest voltage amplitude along this structure. While these changes may be induced by factors such as chronic atrial stretch and chronic atrial arrhythmias, the mechanism of their occurrence in patients with sick sinus syndrome is not known. Pathological studies have suggested that aging itself may be associated with changes within the sinus node [124]. However, the marked contrast in findings between patients with sick sinus syndrome and age-matched controls in this study suggests that they cannot be attributed to the aging process alone [125].

Acknowledgments

This work was funded in part by grants from the National Health and Medical Research Council of Australia and the National Heart Foundation of Australia. Dr Sanders is the recipient of a Medical Postgraduate Research Scholarship from the National Health and Medical Research Council of Australia. Dr Morton is the recipient of a Postgraduate Medical Research Scholarship from the National Heart Foundation of Australia.

References

1 Wijffels MC, Kirchhof CJ, Dorland R, Allessie MA. Atrial fibrillation begets atrial fibrillation. A study in awake chronically instrumented goats. *Circulation* 1995; **92**: 1954–68.

2 Morillo CA, Klein GJ, Jones DL, Guiraudon CM. Chronic rapid atrial pacing. Structural, functional, and electrophysiological characteristics of a new model of sustained atrial fibrillation. *Circulation* 1995; **91**: 1588–95.

3 Gaspo R, Bosch RF, Talajic M, Nattel S. Functional mechanisms underlying tachycardia-induced sustained atrial fibrillation in a chronic dog model. *Circulation* 1997; **96**: 4027–35.

4 Fareh S, Villemaire C, Nattel S. Importance of refractoriness heterogeneity in the enhanced vulnerability to atrial fibrillation induction caused by tachycardia-induced atrial electrical remodeling. *Circulation* 1998; **98**: 2202–9.

5 Morton JB, Byrne MJ, Power JM, Raman J, Kalman JM. Electrical remodeling of the atrium in an anatomic model of atrial flutter: relationship between substrate and triggers for conversion to atrial fibrillation. *Circulation* 2002; **105**: 258–64.

6 Daoud EG, Bogun F, Goyal R *et al*. Effect of atrial fibrillation on atrial refractoriness in humans. *Circulation* 1996; **94**: 1600–6.

7 Kumagai K, Akimitsu S, Kawahira K *et al*. Electrophysiological properties in chronic lone atrial fibrillation. *Circulation* 1991; **84**: 1662–8.

8 Kamalvand K, Tan K, Lloyd G *et al*. Alterations in atrial electrophysiology associated with chronic atrial fibrillation in man. *Eur Heart J* 1999; **20**: 888–95.

9 Franz MR, Karasik PL, Li C, Moubarak J, Chavez M. Electrical remodeling of the human atrium: similar effects in patients with chronic atrial fibrillation and atrial flutter. *J Am Coll Cardiol* 1997; **30**: 1785–92.

10 Sparks PB, Jayaprakash S, Vohra JK, Kalman JM. Electrical remodeling of the atria associated with paroxysmal and chronic atrial flutter. *Circulation* 2000; **102**: 1807–13.

11 Yu WC, Lee SH, Tai CT *et al*. Reversal of atrial electrical remodeling following cardioversion of long-standing atrial fibrillation in man. *Cardiovasc Res* 1999; **42**: 470–6.

12 Elvan A, Wylie K, Zipes DP. Pacing-induced chronic atrial fibrillation impairs sinus node function in dogs. Electrophysiological remodeling. *Circulation* 1996; **94**: 2953–60.

13 Tse HF, Lau CP, Ayers GM. Heterogeneous changes in electrophysiologic properties in the paroxysmal and chronically fibrillating human atrium. *J Cardiovasc Electrophysiol* 1999; **10**: 125–35.

14 Manios EG, Kanoupakis EM, Mavrakis HE *et al.* Sinus pacemaker function after cardioversion of chronic atrial fibrillation: is sinus node remodeling related with recurrence? *J Cardiovasc Electrophysiol* 2001; **12**: 800–6.

15 Daoud EG, Weiss R, Augostini RS *et al.* Remodeling of sinus node function after catheter ablation of right atrial flutter. *J Cardiovasc Electrophysiol* 2002; **13**: 20–4.

16 Luck JC, Engel TR. Dispersion of atrial refractoriness in patients with sinus node dysfunction. *Circulation* 1979; **60**: 404–12.

17 Leistad E, Aksnes G, Verburg E, Christensen G. Atrial contractile dysfunction after short-term atrial fibrillation is reduced by verapamil but increased by BAY K8644. *Circulation* 1996; **93**: 1747–54.

18 Sun H, Gaspo R, Leblanc N, Nattel S. Cellular mechanisms of atrial contractile dysfunction caused by sustained atrial tachycardia. *Circulation* 1998; **98**: 719–27.

19 Yue L, Feng J, Gaspo R *et al.* Ionic remodeling underlying action potential changes in a canine model of atrial fibrillation. *Circ Res* 1997; **81**: 512–25.

20 Bosch RF, Zeng X, Grammer JB, Popovic K, Mewis C, Kuhlkamp V. Ionic mechanisms of electrical remodeling in human atrial fibrillation. *Cardiovasc Res* 1999; **44**: 121–31.

21 Van Wagoner DR, Pond AL, Lamorgese M *et al.* Atrial L-type Ca2+ currents and human atrial fibrillation. *Circ Res* 1999; **85**: 428–36.

22 Brundel BJ, Van Gelder IC, Henning RH *et al.* Ion channel remodeling is related to intraoperative atrial effective refractory periods in patients with paroxysmal and persistent atrial fibrillation. *Circulation* 2001; **103**: 684–90.

23 Schotten U, Ausma J, Stellbrink C *et al.* Cellular mechanisms of depressed atrial contractility in patients with chronic atrial fibrillation. *Circulation* 2001; **103**: 691–8.

24 Tieleman RG, De Langen C, Van Gelder IC *et al.* Verapamil reduces tachycardia-induced electrical remodeling of the atria. *Circulation* 1997; **95**: 1945–53.

25 Fareh S, Benardeau A, Nattel S. Differential efficacy of L- and T-type calcium channel blockers in preventing tachycardia-induced atrial remodeling in dogs. *Cardiovasc Res* 2001; **49**: 762–70.

26 Lee SH, Yu WC, Cheng JJ *et al.* Effect of verapamil on long-term tachycardia-induced atrial electrical remodeling. *Circulation* 2000; **101**: 200–6.

27 Fareh S, Benardeau A, Thibault B, Nattel S. The T-type Ca(2+) channel blocker mibefradil prevents the development of a substrate for atrial fibrillation by tachycardia-induced atrial remodeling in dogs. *Circulation* 1999; **100**: 2191–7.

28 Gaspo R, Bosch RF, Bou-Abboud E, Nattel S. Tachycardia-induced changes in Na+ current in a chronic dog model of atrial fibrillation. *Circ Res* 1997; **81**: 1045–52.

29 Van Wagoner DR, Pond AL, McCarthy PM, Trimmer JS, Nerbonne JM. Outward K+ current densities and Kv1.5 expression are reduced in chronic human atrial fibrillation. *Circ Res* 1997; **80**: 772–81.

30 Allessie M, Ausma J, Schotten U. Electrical, contractile and structural remodeling during atrial fibrillation. *Cardiovasc Res* 2002; **54**: 230–46.

31 Thijssen VL, Ausma J, Liu GS *et al.* Structural changes of atrial myocardium during chronic atrial fibrillation. *Cardiovasc Pathol* 2000; **9**: 17–28.

32 Ausma J, Litjens N, Lenders MH *et al.* Time course of atrial fibrillation-induced cellular structural remodeling in atria of the goat. *J Mol Cell Cardiol* 2001; **33**: 2083–94.

33 Ausma J, Wijffels M, van Eys G, Koide M *et al.* Dedifferentiation of atrial cardiomyocytes as a result of chronic atrial fibrillation. *Am J Pathol* 1997; **151**: 985–97.

34 Mary-Rabine L, Albert A, Pham TD *et al*. The relationship of human atrial cellular electro-physiology to clinical function and ultrastructure. *Circ Res* 1983; **52**: 188–99.

35 Aime-Sempe C, Folliguet T, Rucker-Martin C *et al*. Myocardial cell death in fibrillating and dilated human right atria. *J Am Coll Cardiol* 1999; **34**: 1577–86.

36 Kostin S, Klein G, Szalay Z *et al*. Structural correlate of atrial fibrillation in human patients. *Cardiovasc Res* 2002; **54**: 361–79.

37 Ausma J, van der Velden HMW, Lenders MH *et al*. Reverse structural and gap-junctional remodeling after prolonged atrial fibrillation in the goat. *Circulation* 2003; **107**: 2051–8.

38 Yu WC, Chen SA, Lee SH *et al*. Tachycardia-induced change of atrial refractory period in humans: rate dependency and effects of antiarrhythmic drugs. *Circulation* 1998; **97**: 2331–7.

39 Garratt CJ, Duytschaever M, Killian M *et al*. Repetitive electrical remodeling by paroxysms of atrial fibrillation in the goat: no cumulative effect on inducibility or stability of atrial fibrillation. *J Cardiovasc Electrophysiol* 1999; **10**: 1101–8.

40 Fynn SP, Todd DM, Hobbs WJ *et al*. Clinical evaluation of a policy of early repeated internal cardioversion for recurrence of atrial fibrillation. *J Cardiovasc Electrophysiol* 2002; **13**: 135–41.

41 Rodriguez LM, Timmermans C, Wellens HJ. Are electrophysiological changes induced by longer lasting atrial fibrillation reversible? Observations using the atrial defibrillator. *Circulation* 1999; **100**: 113–16.

42 Ramanna H, Hauer RN, Wittkampf FH *et al*. Identification of the substrate of atrial vulnerability in patients with idiopathic atrial fibrillation. *Circulation* 2000; **101**: 995–1001.

43 Kaseda S, Zipes DP. Contraction-excitation feedback in the atria: a cause of changes in refractoriness. *J Am Coll Cardiol* 1988; **11**: 1327–36.

44 Satoh T, Zipes DP. Unequal atrial stretch in dogs increases dispersion of refractoriness conducive to developing atrial fibrillation. *J Cardiovasc Electrophysiol* 1996; **7**: 833–42.

45 Wijffels MC, Kirchhof CJ, Dorland R, Power J, Allessie MA. Electrical remodeling due to atrial fibrillation in chronically instrumented conscious goats: roles of neurohumoral changes, ischemia, atrial stretch, and high rate of electrical activation. *Circulation* 1997; **96**: 3710–20.

46 Sideris DA, Toumanidis ST, Thodorakis M *et al*. Some observations on the mechanism of pressure related atrial fibrillation. *Eur Heart J* 1994; **15**: 1585–9.

47 Ravelli F, Allessie M. Effects of atrial dilatation on refractory period and vulnerability to atrial fibrillation in the isolated Langendorff-perfused rabbit heart. *Circulation* 1997; **96**: 1686–95.

48 Nazir SA, Lab MJ. Mechanoelectric feedback in the atrium of the isolated guinea-pig heart. *Cardiovasc Res* 1996; **32**: 112–19.

49 Calkins H, el Atassi R, Leon A *et al*. Effect of the atrioventricular relationship on atrial refractoriness in humans. *Pacing Clin Electrophysiol* 1992; **15**: 771–8.

50 Calkins H, el Atassi R, Kalbfleisch S, Langberg J, Morady F. Effects of an acute increase in atrial pressure on atrial refractoriness in humans. *Pacing Clin Electrophysiol* 1992; **15**: 1674–80.

51 Tse HF, Pelosi F, Oral H *et al*. Effects of simultaneous atrioventricular pacing on atrial refractoriness and atrial fibrillation inducibility: role of atrial mechano-electric feedback. *J Cardiovasc Electrophysiol* 2001; **12**: 43–50.

52 Klein LS, Miles WM, Zipes DP. Effect of atrioventricular interval during pacing or recipro-cating tachycardia on atrial size, pressure, and refractory period. Contraction-excitation feedback in human atrium. *Circulation* 1990; **82**: 60–8.

53 Chen YJ, Tai CT, Chiou CW *et al*. Inducibility of atrial fibrillation during atrioventricular pacing with varying intervals: role of atrial electrophysiology and the autonomic nervous system. *J Cardiovasc Electrophysiol* 1999; **10**: 1578–85.

54 Chen YJ, Chen SA, Tai CT *et al*. Role of atrial electrophysiology and autonomic nervous system in patients with supraventricular tachycardia and paroxysmal atrial fibrillation. *J Am Coll Cardiol* 1998; **32**: 732–8.

55 Boyden PA, Hoffman BF. The effects on atrial electrophysiology and structure of surgically induced right atrial enlargement in dogs. *Circ Res* 1981; **49**: 1319–31.

56 Boyden PA, Tilley LP, Pham TD *et al*. Effects of left atrial enlargement on atrial transmembrane potentials and structure in dogs with mitral valve fibrosis. *Am J Cardiol* 1982; **49**: 1896–908.

57 Boyden PA, Tilley LP, Albala A *et al*. Mechanisms for atrial arrhythmias associated with cardiomyopathy: a study of feline hearts with primary myocardial disease. *Circulation* 1984; **69**: 1036–47.

58 Li D, Fareh S, Leung TK, Nattel S. Promotion of atrial fibrillation by heart failure in dogs: atrial remodeling of a different sort. *Circulation* 1999; **100**: 87–95.

59 Shinagawa K, Shi YF, Tardif JC, Leung TK, Nattel S. Dynamic nature of atrial fibrillation substrate during development and reversal of heart failure in dogs. *Circulation* 2002; **105**: 2672–8.

60 Li D, Shinagawa K, Pang L *et al*. Effects of angiotensin-converting enzyme inhibition on the development of the atrial fibrillation substrate in dogs with ventricular tachypacing-induced congestive heart failure. *Circulation* 2001; **104**: 2608–14.

61 Verheule S, Wilson EE, Sih H, Vaz D, Olgin JE. Alteration in atrial electrophysiology due to chronic atrial dilatation in a canine model of mitral regurgitation. *Circulation* 2001; **104** (Suppl II): II-76.

62 Chen YJ, Chen SA, Tai CT *et al*. Electrophysiologic characteristics of a dilated atrium in patients with paroxysmal atrial fibrillation and atrial flutter. *J Interv Card Electrophysiol* 1998; **2**: 181–6.

63 Sparks PB, Mond HG, Vohra JK, Jayaprakash S, Kalman JM. Electrical remodeling of the atria following loss of atrioventricular synchrony: a long-term study in humans. *Circulation* 1999; **100**: 1894–900.

64 Sparks PB, Mond HG, Vohra JK *et al*. Mechanical remodeling of the left atrium after loss of atrioventricular synchrony. A long-term study in humans. *Circulation* 1999; **100**: 1714–21.

65 Willems R, Sipido KR, Holemans P *et al*. Different patterns of angiotensin II and atrial natriuretic peptide secretion in a sheep model of atrial fibrillation. *J Cardiovasc Electrophysiol* 2001; **12**: 1387–92.

66 Everett TH, Li H, Mangrum JM *et al*. Electrical, morphological, and ultrastructural remodeling and reverse remodeling in a canine model of chronic atrial fibrillation. *Circulation* 2000; **102**: 1454–60.

67 Elvan A, Huang XD, Pressler ML, Zipes DP. Radiofrequency catheter ablation of the atria eliminates pacing-induced sustained atrial fibrillation and reduces connexin 43 in dogs. *Circulation* 1997; **96**: 1675–85.

68 van der Velden HM, van Kempen MJ, Wijffels MC *et al*. Altered pattern of connexin40 distribution in persistent atrial fibrillation in the goat. *J Cardiovasc Electrophysiol* 1998; **9**: 596–607.

69 Rocken C, Peters B, Juenemann G *et al*. Atrial amyloidosis. An arrhythmogenic substrate for persistent atrial fibrillation. *Circulation* 2002; **106**: 2091–7.

70 Arndt M, Lendeckel U, Rocken C *et al*. Altered expression of ADAMs (A Disintegrin And Metalloproteinase) in fibrillating human atria. *Circulation* 2002; **105**: 720–5.

71 Nakashima H, Kumagai K, Urata H *et al.* Angiotensin II antagonist prevents electrical remodeling in atrial fibrillation. *Circulation* 2000; **101**: 2612–17.

72 Goette A, Staack T, Rocken C *et al.* Increased expression of extracellular signal-regulated kinase and angiotensin-converting enzyme in human atria during atrial fibrillation. *J Am Coll Cardiol* 2000; **35**: 1669–77.

73 Goette A, Arndt M, Rocken C *et al.* Regulation of angiotensin II receptor subtypes during atrial fibrillation in humans. *Circulation* 2000; **101**: 2678–81.

74 Wolf PA, Kannel WB, McGee DL *et al.* Duration of atrial fibrillation and imminence of stroke: the Framingham study. *Stroke* 1983; **14**: 664–7.

75 Wolf PA, Abbott RD, Kannel WB. Atrial fibrillation as an independent risk factor for stroke: the Framingham Study. *Stroke* 1991; **22**: 983–8.

76 Wolf PA, Dawber TR, Thomas HE Jr, Kannel WB. Epidemiologic assessment of chronic atrial fibrillation and risk of stroke: the Framingham study. *Neurology* 1978; **28**: 973–7.

77 Ezekowitz MD, James KE, Nazarian SM *et al.* Silent cerebral infarction in patients with nonrheumatic atrial fibrillation. The Veterans Affairs Stroke Prevention in Nonrheumatic Atrial Fibrillation Investigators. *Circulation* 1995; **92**: 2178–82.

78 Lin HJ, Wolf PA, Kelly-Hayes M *et al.* Stroke severity in atrial fibrillation. The Framingham Study. *Stroke* 1996; **27**: 1760–4.

79 Manning WJ, Silverman DI, Katz SE, Douglas PS. Atrial ejection force: a noninvasive assessment of atrial systolic function. *J Am Coll Cardiol* 1993; **22**: 221–5.

80 Grimm RA, Stewart WJ, Maloney JD *et al.* Impact of electrical cardioversion for atrial fibrillation on left atrial appendage function and spontaneous echo contrast: characterization by simultaneous transesophageal echocardiography. *J Am Coll Cardiol* 1993; **22**: 1359–66.

81 Pollick C, Taylor D. Assessment of left atrial appendage function by transesophageal echocardiography. Implications for the development of thrombus. *Circulation* 1991; **84**: 223–31.

82 Sparks PB, Jayaprakash S, Vohra JK *et al.* Left atrial 'stunning' following radiofrequency catheter ablation of chronic atrial flutter. *J Am Coll Cardiol* 1998; **32**: 468–75.

83 Welch PJ, Afridi I, Joglar JA *et al.* Effect of radiofrequency ablation on atrial mechanical function in patients with atrial flutter. *Am J Cardiol* 1999; **84**: 420–5.

84 Grimm RA, Stewart WJ, Arheart K, Thomas JD, Klein AL. Left atrial appendage 'stunning' after electrical cardioversion of atrial flutter: an attenuated response compared with atrial fibrillation as the mechanism for lower susceptibility to thromboembolic events. *J Am Coll Cardiol* 1997; **29**: 582–9.

85 Goldman MJ. The management of chronic atrial fibrillation. *Prog Cardiovasc Dis* 1960; **2**: 465–79.

86 Black IW, Fatkin D, Sagar KB *et al.* Exclusion of atrial thrombus by transesophageal echocardiography does not preclude embolism after cardioversion of atrial fibrillation. A multicenter study. *Circulation* 1994; **89**: 2509–513.

87 Falk RH. Atrial fibrillation. *N Engl J Med* 2001; **344**: 1067–78.

88 Fuster V, Ryden LE, Asinger RW *et al.* ACC/AHA/ESC guidelines for the management of patients with atrial fibrillation: executive summary a report of the American College of Cardiology/American Heart Association Task Force on Practice Guidelines and the European Society of Cardiology Committee for Practice Guidelines and Policy Conferences (Committee to Develop Guidelines for the Management of Patients With Atrial Fibrillation) developed in collaboration with the North American Society of Pacing and Electrophysiology. *Circulation* 2001; **104**: 2118–50.

89 Louie EK, Liu D, Reynertson SI *et al.* 'Stunning' of the left atrium after spontaneous conversion of atrial fibrillation to sinus rhythm: demonstration by transesophageal Doppler techniques in a canine model. *J Am Coll Cardiol* 1998; **32**: 2081–6.

90 Altemose GT, Zipes DP, Weksler J, Miller JM, Olgin JE. Inhibition of the Na(+)/H(+) exchanger delays the development of rapid pacing-induced atrial contractile dysfunction. *Circulation* 2001; **103**: 762–8.

91 Schotten U, Duytschaever M, Ausma J *et al.* Electrical and contractile remodeling during the first days of atrial fibrillation go hand in hand. *Circulation* 2003; **107**: 1433–9.

92 Daoud EG, Marcovitz P, Knight BP *et al.* Short-term effect of atrial fibrillation on atrial contractile function in humans. *Circulation* 1999; **99**: 3024–7.

93 Sparks PB, Jayaprakash S, Mond HG *et al.* Left atrial mechanical function after brief duration atrial fibrillation. *J Am Coll Cardiol* 1999; **33**: 342–9.

94 Harjai K, Mobarek S, Abi-Samra F *et al.* Mechanical dysfunction of the left atrium and the left atrial appendage following cardioversion of atrial fibrillation and its relation to total electrical energy used for cardioversion. *Am J Cardiol* 1998; **81**: 1125–9.

95 Dodds GA III, Wilkinson WE, Greenfield RA *et al.* Evaluation of the effect of transthoracic cardioversion from ventricular tachycardia to sinus rhythm on left atrial mechanical function. *Am J Cardiol* 1996; **78**: 1436–9.

96 Sparks PB, Kulkarni R, Vohra JK *et al.* Effect of direct current shocks on left atrial mechanical function in patients with structural heart disease. *J Am Coll Cardiol* 1998; **31**: 1395–9.

97 Antonielli E, Pizzuti A, Bassignana A *et al.* Transesophageal echocardiographic evidence of more pronounced left atrial stunning after chemical (propafenone) rather than electrical attempts at cardioversion from atrial fibrillation. *Am J Cardiol* 1999; **84**: 1092–110.

98 Grimm RA, Leung DY, Black IW *et al.* Left atrial appendage 'stunning' after spontaneous conversion of atrial fibrillation demonstrated by transesophageal Doppler echocardiography. *Am Heart J* 1995; **130**: 174–6.

99 Jordaens L, Missault L, Germonpre E *et al.* Delayed restoration of atrial function after conversion of atrial flutter by pacing or electrical cardioversion. *Am J Cardiol* 1993; **71**: 63–7.

100 Weiss R, Marcovitz P, Knight BP *et al.* Acute changes in spontaneous echo contrast and atrial function after cardioversion of persistent atrial flutter. *Am J Cardiol* 1998; **82**: 1052–5.

101 Mulieri LA, Hasenfuss G, Leavitt B, Allen PD, Alpert NR. Altered myocardial force-frequency relation in human heart failure. *Circulation* 1992; **85**: 1743–50.

102 Bers DM. Calcium fluxes involved in control of cardiac myocyte contraction. *Circ Res* 2000; **87**: 275–81.

103 Brixius K, Pietsch M, Schwinger RH. The intracellular Ca(2+)-homeostasis influences the frequency-dependent force-generation in man. *Basic Res Cardiol* 1999; **94**: 152–8.

104 Hasenfuss G, Reinecke H, Studer R *et al.* Relation between myocardial function and expression of sarcoplasmic reticulum Ca(2+)-ATPase in failing and nonfailing human myocardium. *Circ Res* 1994; **75**: 434–42.

105 Yard NJ, Chiesi M, Ball HA. Effect of cyclopiazonic acid, an inhibitor of sarcoplasmic reticulum Ca(2+)-ATPase, on the frequency-dependence of the contraction-relaxation cycle of the guinea-pig isolated atrium. *Br J Pharmacol* 1994; **113**: 1001–7.

106 Sanders P, Morton JB, Morgan JG *et al.* Reversal of atrial mechanical stunning after cardioversion of atrial arrhythmias. Implications for the mechanisms of tachycardia mediated atrial cardiomyopathy. *Circulation* 2002; **106**: 1806–13.

107 Schotten U, Greiser M, Benke D *et al.* Atrial fibrillation-induced atrial contractile dysfunction: a tachycardiomyopathy of a different sort. *Cardiovasc Res* 2002; **53**: 192–201.

108 Ausma J, Wijffels M, Thone F *et al.* Structural changes of atrial myocardium due to sustained atrial fibrillation in the goat. *Circulation* 1997; **96**: 3157–63.

109 Sanders P, Morton JB, Kistler PM *et al.* Reversal of atrial mechanical dysfunction in humans with atrial fibrillation: implications for the mechanisms of atrial mechanical remodeling. *Circulation* 2002; **106** (Suppl II): 189.

110 Mondillo S, Sabatini L, Agricola E *et al.* Correlation between left atrial size, prothrombotic state and markers of endothelial dysfunction in patients with lone chronic nonrheumatic atrial fibrillation. *Int J Cardiol* 2000; **75**: 227–32.

111 Brundel BJJM, Van Gelder IC, Tuinenburg AE *et al.* Endothelin system in human persistent and paroxysmal atrial fibrillation. *J Cardiovasc Electrophysiol* 2001; **12**: 737–42.

112 Cai H, Li Z, Goette A *et al.* Downregulation of endocardial nitric oxide synthase expression and nitric oxide production in atrial fibrillation. Potential mechanisms for atrial thrombosis and stroke. *Circulation* 2002; **106**: 2854–8.

113 Tieleman RG, Van Gelder IC, Brundel BJJM *et al.* Mitral regurgitation is associated with prolongation of the atrial refractory period. *Circulation* 2002; **106** (Suppl II): II-370.

114 Fan K, Lee KL, Chow WH, Chau E, Lau CP. Internal cardioversion of chronic atrial fibrillation during percutaneous mitral commissurotomy: insight into reversal of chronic stretch-induced atrial remodeling. *Circulation* 2002; **105**: 2746–52.

115 Sanders P, Morton JB, Davidson NC *et al.* Electrical remodeling of the atria in heart failure: electrophysiologic and electroanatomic mapping to determine the substrate for atrial fibrillation in humans. *Circulation* 2003; **108**: 1461–8.

116 Ohtani K, Yutani C, Nagata S *et al.* High prevalence of atrial fibrosis in patients with dilated cardiomyopathy. *J Am Coll Cardiol* 1995; **25**: 1162–9.

117 Morton JB, Sanders P, Vohra JK *et al.* The effect of chronic atrial stretch on atrial electrical remodeling in patients with an atrial septal defect. *Circulation* 2003; **107**: 1775–82.

118 Liu Z, Hayano M, Hirata T *et al.* Abnormalities of electrocardiographic P wave morphology and their relation to electrophysiological parameters of the atrium in patients with sick sinus syndrome. *Pacing Clin Electrophysiol* 1998; **21**: 79–86.

119 Tanigawa M, Fukatani M, Konoe A *et al.* Prolonged and fractionated right atrial electrograms during sinus rhythm in patients with paroxysmal atrial fibrillation and sick sinus node syndrome. *J Am Coll Cardiol* 1991; **17**: 403–8.

120 Centurion OA, Isomoto S, Fukatani M *et al.* Relationship between atrial conduction defects and fractionated atrial endocardial electrograms in patients with sick sinus syndrome. *Pacing Clin Electrophysiol* 1993; **16**: 2022–33.

121 Centurion OA, Fukatani M, Konoe A *et al.* Different distribution of abnormal endocardial electrograms within the right atrium in patients with sick sinus syndrome. *Br Heart J* 1992; **68**: 596–600.

122 De Sisti A, Leclercq JF, Fiorello P *et al.* Electrophysiologic characteristics of the atrium in sinus node dysfunction: atrial refractoriness and conduction. *J Cardiovasc Electrophysiol* 2000; **11**: 30–3.

123 Sanders P, Morton JB, Kistler PM *et al.* Electrophysiologic and electroanatomic characterization of the atria in sinus node disease: evidence of diffuse atrial remodeling. *J Am Coll Cardiol* 2003; **41** (Suppl A): 121A.

124 Lev M. Aging changes in the human sinoatrial node. *J Gerontol* 1954; **9**: 1–9.

125 Allessie MA, Boyden PA, Camm AJ *et al.* Pathophysiology and prevention of atrial fibrillation. *Circulation* 2001; **103**: 769–77.

PART II

Developing Strategies for AF Management

CHAPTER 6

Atrioventricular Node Ablation

J. David Burkhardt, Bruce L. Wilkoff

In this chapter we review atrioventricular (AV) node ablation with permanent pacemaker insertion ('ablate and pace'), which was first proposed as an atrial fibrillation (AF) therapy in 1982 by Gallagher *et al.* [1]. The purpose of the procedure is to electrically isolate ventricular electrical activation from chaotic and rapid atrial activation; this allows the ventricle to contract at a regular programmed rate. Initially, direct current energy was used to ablate the AV node, requiring general anesthesia and introducing risks, including barotrauma. However, the current art of radiofrequency energy-based ablation is technically straightforward and widely practiced.

Procedure outcome

The rate of success in achieving complete AV block is very high. According to the North American Society of Pacing and Electrophysiology (NASPE) Prospective Voluntary Registry, the success rate for AV node ablation was 97.4% [2]. No significant differences were noted when comparing large-volume centers with lower-volume centers or teaching and non-teaching institutions. In the Ablate and Pace Trial, the rate was 99.4% [3]. This percentage includes 3% of patients who required a second ablation procedure after early recovery of AV node conduction.

In patients with refractory atrial fibrillation, several studies have demonstrated patient benefit after ablate and pace. In the Ablate and Pace Trial, patients experienced improved quality of life and diminished symptoms, as well as an increase in left ventricular ejection fraction if it was depressed prior to the procedure [3]. Brignole and colleagues performed a multicenter, randomized trial comparing ablate and pace to pharmacotherapy in patients with heart failure or other severe symptoms, structural heart disease, and a resting heart rate greater than ninety beats per minute [4]. This study of 66 patients revealed superior symptom improvement in the ablate and pace group. No increase in left ventricular ejection fraction or exercise capacity was noted. To exclude the possibility of placebo effect in implanting a permanent pacemaker, Natale *et al.* studied patients with persistent AF that was pharmacologically well rate-controlled at rest and with exercise [5]. He divided the patients into three groups. The first group underwent ablate and pace with discontinuation of pharmacotherapy. The second group underwent ablate and pace without discontinuation of pharmacotherapy, and the third group underwent pacemaker implantation without AV node ablation and without discontinuation of continued pharmacotherapy. The groups that underwent AV node ablation experienced improved symptoms and quality of life, although the first group had a more dramatic response. There was no improvement in the third group. A small increase in the left ventricular ejection fraction was seen in the first group only. No group demonstrated increased exercise duration. A recent meta-analysis of 21 ablate and pace studies totaling 1181 patients revealed significant improvement in quality of life measures, exercise duration, left ventricular ejection fraction, in association with a significant reduction in health-care utilization [6]. The risks of AV junction ablation are low and frequently related to the pacemaker insertion. In the NASPE registry, only five significant complications occurred in 646 patients [2]. The incidence of complications did not vary with center volume or whether the institution was a teaching facility or not. In the Ablate and Pace Trial, seven of 156 patients experienced early complications, which included lead dislodgment requiring repositioning in two patients, and pacemaker pocket hematoma, hemopneumothorax requiring thoracostomy tube drainage, femoral vein thrombosis, and transient hypotension in one patient each. Late complications occurred in 5.1% of patients, including stroke in four patients, lead malfunction in two patients, and non-sustained ventricular tachycardia in one patient [3]. Of particular concern was the incidence of sudden death in this trial, which was 9% during the first year after the procedure; factors associated with sudden death included left ventricular systolic dysfunction and congestive heart failure. A European registry also reported torsade des pointes and sudden death at a low frequency [7]. It is worth noting that the period encompassed by these data preceded the recognition of the need for high rate pacing to prevent pleomorphic ventricular tachycardia, particularly early after the procedure. In trials which included a control (non-ablation) group, no significant increase in the rate of sudden death has been observed [4, 5, 8–12]. In the meta-analysis, total and sudden death mortalities were comparable with medical therapy [6].

In patients with symptomatic AF, ablate and pace is probably quite cost-effective, given subsequent reductions in pharmacotherapy and health-care utilization relative to unrelated evaluations of pharmacotherapy [13–15]. However, appropriately controlled prospective studies have yet to be reported.

Current use

Ablate and pace is used primarily as a therapy of last resort to diminish AF symptoms in patients with rapid ventricular response. The NASPE registry reported that of 3357 patients who received catheter ablation procedures, 646 were for AV junction ablation [2]. In 1993, 2.5% of permanent pacemakers were placed for AV junction ablation [16]. At the Cleveland Clinic in 2001, 40 AV junction ablation procedures were performed out of more than 700 total ablation procedures and more than 4000 electrophysiological procedures. In view of the incidence of AF, these data are consistent with the notion that the procedure is used infrequently. A recent report of ablate and pace typifies the current ablate and pace patient: symptoms for 6.4 ± 3.5 years, multiple hospital admissions, failure or intolerance of multiple antiarrhythmic drugs, and a mean NYHA class of 2.7 ± 0.6 [13]. The hesitancy to use this procedure comes from both practitioners and patients, given its irreversible nature and the subsequent device dependence. For these reasons, it is much more commonly performed in the elderly. Given the typical demographic and previous reports demonstrating an association with sudden death, and in view of recent concerns regarding the introduction of mechanical dyssynchrony by right ventricular pacing, at present there is also significant hesitation in performing this procedure in patients with systolic dysfunction.

The hesitation to use ablate and pace is of interest when viewed in the context of the recent explosion in cardiac resynchronization therapy (CRT), which also renders patients pacemaker-dependent. The annual frequency of CRT device implantation far surpasses ablate and pace procedures at the Cleveland Clinic, yet the data in support of these therapies are very similar [17, 18].

Ablate and pace in context

There would be little argument against atrial rhythm control if a 'magic wand' therapy (one that is completely safe and efficacious) were at hand. However, the fact that such a therapy does not currently and may never exist calls for evolution away from an all-or-none therapy paradigm. Apart from cardio-embolism, AF can be deconstructed into four distinct problems: (i) elevated ventricular rate; (ii) irregular ventricular rhythm; (iii) loss of atrial mechanical contribution; and (iv) other mischief imposed by the fibrillating atria. Ventricular rate is the only problem which has been consistently demonstrated in man to have significant physiological repercussions [19]. It is reasonable to think of ablate and pace as perfect ventricular rate control. In recent years, multiple studies have confirmed that (largely pharmacological) ventricular rate control plus warfarin anticoagulation is equivalent or superior to pharmacological atrial rhythm control [18, 20]. No studies have directly compared ablate and pace with non-pharmacological atrial rhythm control strategies.

The future of ablate and pace

We believe that the future of ablate and pace is bright. This is based on four considerations. First, the prevalence of AF is expected to increase markedly in the coming decades, in association with the increasing age demographic and incidence of hypertension and obesity, and improved survival of patients with cardiovascular comorbidity. It is critical to understand that AF is a disease of the elderly. Secondly, we have reservations as to the future of therapies for atrial rhythm control, particularly in the elderly. Pharmacotherapy is clearly unacceptable as a long-term strategy, given the issues of inefficacy, intolerance, risk and cost [21, 22]. Device-based atrial rhythm control is beset by similar issues. Ablation therapy is immature and evolving; successful, long-term AF suppression is clearly possible. However, success rates in patients with persistent AF have been disappointing, complication rates have been significant, and the frailty factor in the typical AF patient may prohibit broad application. Thirdly, pharmacological rate control is suboptimal, primarily due to intolerance when strictly applied. In addition to more front-line use as a therapy to ameliorate symptoms, we feel that ablate and pace will also find increasing use as a means of stabilizing or reversing diminished left ventricular systolic function in the setting of high ventricular rates, independently of symptoms [19]. Fourthly, the motivation to pursue atrial rhythm control in order to remove anticoagulants will probably wane. Certainly, warfarin is a major problem for many patients, because of compliance, morbidity and inconvenience. However, recent studies have emphasized that the removal of warfarin in association with a rhythm control strategy is unwise [18]. Evaluations of pharmacotherapies to replace warfarin are in progress, including thrombin inhibitors [23]. Non-pharmacological strategies to eliminate AF-attributable cardioembolic risk are also in development [24]; if efficacy can be demonstrated at a low level of risk, this therapy combined with ablate and pace may represent a 'curative' option for a more representative AF demographic.

The specifics of the pacing technique used in ablate and pace will probably evolve. Recent studies have suggested that the ventricular electromechanical activation sequence (dyssynchrony) associated with right ventricular pacing undermines left ventricular function, which may have serious clinical repercussions [25]. Diminishment in left ventricular systolic function is a well-described entity after ablate and pace, albeit rare [19, 26]. The infrequency of this phenomenon is probably due in part to the historical selection of patients with persistent rapid ventricular response, the amelioration of which probably dominates any adverse impact of dyssynchrony. Certainly, future expanded use of ablate and pace in patients without persistent rapid ventricular response will require a re-examination of this issue, particularly in patients with compromised left ventricular systolic function. Recent reports have suggested that CRT can prevent or reverse left ventricular dysfunction associated with right ventricular pacing [26–29]. Interestingly, these studies have also called into question the benefit of AF suppression in the setting of complete heart block and CRT [28].

In summary, it is clear that ablate and pace is a very effective therapy for symptom control in patients with atrial fibrillation. Outcomes with this therapy have highlighted the potential for high ventricular rate (and irregularity?) to degrade left ventricular mechanical function. The procedure is high-success, low-risk and probably quite cost-effective. Although the specific pacing technique will evolve, the central concept (ventricular rate and regularity control) is mature. Given these features, we would propose that ablate and pace form the gold standard against which any non-pharmacological therapy for atrial rhythm control should be directly compared. In addition, we would propose that studies be performed to demonstrate whether there is any additional benefit in atrial rhythm control in the setting of ablate and CRT.

References

1 Gallagher JJ, Svenson RH, Kasell JH *et al.* Catheter technique for closed-chest ablation of the atrioventricular conduction system. *N Engl J Med* 1982; **306**: 194–200.

2 Scheinman MM, Huang S. The 1998 NASPE prospective catheter ablation registry. *Pacing Clin Electrophysiol* 2000; **23**: 1020–8.

3 Kay GN, Ellenbogen KA, Giudici M. The Ablate and Pace Trial: a prospective study of catheter ablation of the AV conduction system and permanent pacemaker implantation for the treatment of atrial fibrillation. *J Interv Card Electrophysiol* 1998; **2**: 121–35.

4 Brignole M, Menozzi C, Gianfranchi L *et al.* Assessment of atrioventricular junction ablation and VVIR pacemaker versus pharmacological treatment in patients with heart failure and chronic atrial fibrillation: a randomized, controlled study. *Circulation* 1998; **98**: 953–60.

5 Natale A, Zimmerman L, Tomassoni G *et al.* AV node ablation and pacemaker implantation after withdrawal of effective rate-control medications for chronic atrial fibrillation: effect on quality of life and exercise performance. *Pacing Clin Electrophysiol* 1999; **22**: 1634–9.

6 Wood MA, Brown-Mahoney C, Kay GN *et al.* Clinical outcomes after ablation and pacing therapy for atrial fibrillation: a meta-analysis. *Circulation* 2000; **101**: 1138–44.

7 Hindricks G, on behalf of the Multicentre European Radiofrequency Survey (MERFS). The Multicentre European Radiofrequency Survey (MERFS): complications of radiofrequency catheter ablation of arrhythmias. *Eur Heart J* 1993; **14**: 1644–53.

8 Evans GT, Scheinman MM, and the Executive Committee of the Registry. The percutaneous cardiac mapping and ablation registry: summary of results. *PACE* 1987; **10**: 1395–9.

9 Evans GT, Scheinman MM, Bardy G *et al.* Predictors of in hospital mortality after DC catheter ablation of atrioventricular junction: results of a prospective, international, multi-center study. *Circulation* 1991; **84**: 1924–37.

10 Auricchio A, Klein H, Trappe HJ *et al.* Effect on ventricular performance of direct current electrical shock for catheter ablation of the atrioventricular junction. *PACE* 1992; **15**: 344–56.

11 Brignole M, Menozzi C, Gianfranchi L *et al.* An assessment of atrioventricular junction ablation and DDDR mode-switching pacemaker versus pharmacological treatment in patients with severely symptomatic paroxysmal atrial fibrillation: a randomized controlled study. *Circulation* 1997; **96**: 2617–24.

12 Ozcan C, Jahangir A, Friedman PA *et al.* Long-term survival after ablation of the atrioventricular node and implantation of permanent pacemaker in patients with atrial fibrillation. *N Engl J Med* 2001; **344**: 1043–51.

13 Manolis AG, Katsivas AG, Lazaris EE *et al.* Ventricular performance and quality of life in patients who underwent radiofrequency AV junction ablation and permanent pacemaker implantation due to medically refractory atrial tachyarrhythmias. *J Interv Card Electrophysiol* 1998; **2**: 71–6.

14 Jensen S, Bergfeldt L, Rosenqvist M. Long-term follow-up of patients treated by radiofrequency ablation of the atrioventricular junction. *PACE* 1995; **18**: 1609–14.

15 Fitzpatrick A, Kourouyan H, Siu A *et al.* Quality of life and outcomes after radiofrequency his-bundle catheter ablation and permanent pacemaker implantation: impact of treatment in paroxysmal and established atrial fibrillation. *Am Heart J* 1996; **131**: 499–507.

16 Bernstein AD, Parsonnet V. Survey of cardiac pacing and defibrillation in the United States in 1993. *Am J Cardiol* 1996; **78**: 187–96.

17 Abraham WT Fisher WG, Smith AL *et al.*, for the MIRACLE Study Group. Cardiac resynchronization in chronic heart failure. *N Engl J Med* 2002; **346**: 1845–53.

18 Lim HS, Hamaad A, Lip GY. Clinical management of atrial fibrillation-rate versus rhythm control. *Crit Care* 2004; **8**: 217–19

19 Ozcan C, Jahangir A, Friedman PA *et al.* Significant effects of atrioventricular node ablation and pacemaker implantation on left ventricular function and long-term survival in patients with atrial fibrillation and left ventricular dysfunction. *Am J Cardiol* 2003; **92**: 33–7.

20 The Atrial Fibrillation Follow-up Investigation of Rhythm Management (AFFIRM) Investigators. A comparison of rate control and rhythm control in patients with atrial fibrillation. *N Engl J Med* 2002; **347**: 1825–33.

21 Coplen SE, Antmann EM, Berlin JA *et al.* Efficacy and safety of quinidine therapy for maintenance of sinus rhythm after cardioversion: a meta-analysis of randomized control trials. *Circulation* 1990; **82**: 1106–16.

22 Falk RH. Flecainide-induced ventricular tachycardia and fibrillation in patients treated for atrial fibrillation. *Ann Intern Med* 1989; **111**: 107–11.

23 Sinnaeve PR, Van de Werf FJ. Will oral antithrombin agents replace warfarin? *Heart* 2004; **90**: 827–8.

24 Hanna IR, Kolm P, Martine R, Reisman M, Gray W, Block PC. Left atrial structure and function after percutaneous left atrial appendage catheter occlusion (PLAATO): six-month echocardiographic followup. *J Am Coll Cardiol* 2004; **43**: 1868–72.

25 Wilkoff BL, Dual Chamber and VVI Implantable Defibrillator Trial Investigators. The dual chamber and VVI implantable defibrillator (DAVID) trial: rationale, design, results and clinical implications. *Card Electrophysiol Rev* 2003; **4**: 468–72.

26 Nunez A, Alberca MT, Cosio FG *et al.* Severe mitral regurgitation with right ventricular pacing, successfully treated with left ventricular pacing. *Pacing Clin Electrophysiol* 2002; **25**: 226–30.

27 Leclercq C, Walker S, Linde C *et al.* Comparative effects of permanent biventricular and right univentricular pacing in heart failure patients with atrial fibrillation. *Eur Heart J* 2002; **23**: 1780–7.

28 Leon AR, Greenberg JM, Kanuru N *et al.* Cardiac resynchronization in patients with heart failure and chronic atrial fibrillation: effect of upgrading to biventricular pacing after chronic right ventricular pacing. *J Am Coll Cardiol* 2002; **39**: 1258–63.

29 Blanc JJ, Etiene Y, Gilard M. Assessment of left ventricular pacing in patients with severe cardiac failure after atrioventricular node ablation and right ventricular pacing for permanent atrial fibrillation. *Europace* 1999; **1**: 47–8.

CHAPTER 7

Percutaneous Atrial Catheter Ablation

Dipen Shah, Pierre Jais, Michel Haissaguerre

Cox and his colleagues demonstrated the feasibility of eliminating atrial fibrillation (AF) by extensive surgical sectioning of both atria [1]. The early results of catheter-based interventions attempting to imitate surgical efforts were meager because the ablation catheter is ill-suited to duplicating surgical atriotomies. However, the electrophysiological data obtained during the course of these attempts focused attention on the role of the atrial myocardium ensheathing the pulmonary veins [2]. Catheter-based techniques were developed to neutralize the arrhythmogenicity of the pulmonary veins, and adjunctive ablation techniques are at present being evaluated in an effort to include a wider spectrum of patients with AF. In this chapter, we will summarize the past, detail the present, and speculate about the future of percutaneous catheter ablation of AF.

Pulmonary vein ablation

Pulmonary vein anatomy

The pulmonary veins are formed by the confluence of venules originating at the lung periphery, containing little muscle, joining to form larger veins coursing toward the hilum. The venous wall (like that of other veins) consists of a thin endothelium, an irregular media of smooth muscle and fibrous tissue and a thick fibrous adventitia. Near their anatomical junction with the left atrium, sleeves of atrial myocardium extend irregularly into the venous adventitia. The length and coverage of these sleeves of striated myocardium varies from species to species. In rats, dogs and pigs, it is more extensive than in humans, reaching the hilum and even intrapulmonary segments. In human subjects, myocardial extensions are present in all the veins, though the sleeves are more extensive around the superior than around the inferior pulmonary veins and thin out or even disappear as the veins divide into segmental branches. A network of vasa vasorum is present in the muscle layer, along with numerous ganglia, nerve fibers and nerve endings, particularly at the venoatrial junction. While node-like cells (of myocardial origin) have been described in the rat pulmonary vein, recent data from human subjects could not corroborate this finding. Like atrial myocardium in general, the fiber arrangement of this myocardial sleeve is thought to play an important role in determining its electrophysiological properties. Circular or spirally oriented bundles of myocytes interconnect with each other and with other longitudinally or obliquely oriented fibers [3]. Variations are present from vein to vein, and may be related to the branching pattern. Fibrous gaps within these myocardial sleeves are also seen, with a suggestion that they may be more common with advancing age or in the presence of structural heart disease. Common orifices may be found in about 20% of hearts, while an extra orifice (typically in the right middle position) may be detectable in about 10%, though it is important to note that these data have been derived from autopsy specimens and not from clinical imaging data with different definitions for each. The more distal (towards the lungs) portion of the veins serves a conduit-like and capacitative function, and may exhibit vasomotion under appropriate conditions in animal species. A throttle valve or sphincter function of the striated muscle sleeve protecting the lungs from left atrial back pressure and pulmonary edema has been speculated upon.

Pulmonary vein embryology

There are no morphological landmarks during early development which delineate the boundaries of the embryonic venous sinus from the atrial component of the primary heart tube. It is therefore difficult to decide the origin of the pulmonary vein. Recent evidence suggests that the pulmonary vein develops from the mesoderm between the inflow portion of the heart tube and the lung buds that evaginate from the foregut into somatic mesoderm. The surrounds of the pulmonary pit within the embryonic systemic venous sinus discrete from its horns probably develop into the pulmonary veins [4].

Pulmonary vein imaging

The variations in pulmonary vein anatomy from individual to individual and from vein to vein include differences in size, ostial takeoff, and branching pattern. Apart from the fact that superior pulmonary veins have longer muscle sleeves, other anatomical variants, such as common ostia, simply have approximately twice the circumference and therefore may require more extensive ablation. Variants such as extra ostia are clinically important as well, since their myocardial investiture demands specific ablation. A case report of an arrhythmogenic pulmonary vein aneurysm suggests the importance of such anatomical malformations. Echocardiography is unique in providing real-time imaging of the anatomy but has a lower resolution than other techniques, such as angiography, computed tomography and magnetic resonance imaging. Transesophageal echocardiography does a better job of imaging the pulmonary veins than transthoracic echocardiography, though the right inferior pulmonary vein may still be difficult to visualize adequately. Though the exact definition of the venoatrial junction has not been agreed upon, intracardiac echocardiography provides the best visualization of this area. Imaging of the pulmonary veins using intracardiac echocardiography from a probe positioned within the right atrium is frequently inadequate, and thus necessitates positioning the probe in the left atrium through another trans-septal sheath. These probes also have limited or no steerability and lack end-on viewing ability. However, some groups use it routinely for facilitating trans-septal puncture and others for detecting tissue overheating by imaging microbubbles. Angiography can easily be integrated into an electrophysiology study or an ablation procedure and can be repeated as necessary during a procedure to look for acute changes but requires a contrast medium load, which can be problematic in patients with iodine allergies or significant hemodynamic/renal impairment. However, proper technique remains important in optimizing the yield of information using this technique. Pulmonary artery injections followed through the left atrial phase do not achieve sufficient definition of the anatomy even with digital subtraction, and overlapping branches and flow across the mitral valve render interpretation difficult. Selective angiography provides better results but the quality of opacification depends upon contrast concentration, and therefore varies with cardiac output as well as the delivery catheter lumen and tip hole sizes. Since contrast injection during selective pulmonary venography is performed against the direction of blood flow, side branches or nearby ostia may not be opacified, particularly with endhole catheters, and the only indication of the presence of side branches may be a negative shadow of unopacified blood. In order to better identify common ostia, simultaneous contrast injection through two long sheaths or catheters has been proposed (personal communication, A. Takahashi, 2002). A test shot with a small volume of dye is useful to confirm catheter position and to avoid injecting with a wedged catheter tip, which may produce segmental pulmonary edema or consolidation. A bolus of 10–15 ml of contrast (hand injection being safest) is usually necessary in adults to provide proper opacification. The trans-septal sheath itself (8 French) can be conveniently used to opacify the two superior pulmonary veins, and can be guided into the left inferior pulmonary vein over a deflectable ablation catheter to allow contrast injection on withdrawing the ablation catheter. However, the right inferior pulmonary veins can be difficult to cannulate, particularly if they have a low ostium and an upward takeoff. In this situation, a soft 6 French multipurpose angiography catheter can be looped across the left atrium to selectively engage this vein. However, careful attention must be paid during this maneuver to avoid perforating the left atrial appendage. Indeed, the anatomical location of the appendage means that it can easily be mistaken for the left superior pulmonary vein, and incautious advancement of a catheter in this position can perforate this structure, resulting in tamponade. The characteristic swinging contractile movement of the left atrial appendage contrasts with the immobility of the non-contractile and extracardiac pulmonary veins and can be a helpful clue. Both computed tomography (CT) and magnetic resonance (MR) imaging have been successfully used to image the veins before and after the procedure. Their non-invasive nature and their ability to provide multidimensional coverage are significant advantages and render them ideal for preprocedural planning as well as subsequent follow-up. It is unclear if there is any significant advantage of one over the other technique, though the functional potential of MR imaging is alluring. MR imaging cannot be performed in general in patients with pacemakers or even some metallic implants; therefore, CT scans may be the only possible option in these patients. On the other hand MR imaging can avoid an intravenous radiocontrast medium load in patients with hemodynamic or renal impairment, as well as radiation exposure. The main information to be obtained from any imaging study is vein diameter and the number and location of the vein ostia, though intracardiac echo can in addition provide information about catheter contact. When using mapping systems which rely on catheter entry into the requisite structure for reconstructing the anatomy, it is important that the operator should not miss any ostia; properly performed selective angiography will demonstrate closely adjacent ostia, and of course CT or MR scans will certainly show all pulmonary vein ostia. With the advent of mapping devices adapted to the pulmonary vein (circular loop catheters and basket catheters), appropriate sizing and positioning have become increasingly relevant. Vein takeoff angle, ostial size and branching pattern are all important for proper deployment. Commonly used circumferential loop and basket catheters cannot change their deployed diameter (though variable diameter loop catheters are presently being tested), and therefore appropriate sizing is necessary. Very early branching, as is common with the right inferior pulmonary vein, results in an unstable catheter predominantly within the left atrium.

Pulmonary vein electrophysiology

As opposed to smooth muscle, myocardium in the pulmonary veins is known to be electrically active. This myocardium is proximally continuous with the left atrium and distally peters out within a couple of centimeters of the venoatrial junction or in proximity to the first-order branches. Accordingly, activation in sinus rhythm enters from the venoatrial junction and dies out distally, resembling a dead end (cul de sac). On the other hand, during ectopy originating from a particular vein, venous activation precedes adjacent atrial activation. Changing fiber direction, fibrosis and the pathological effects of left heart disease can all result in delayed activation – manifest as fractionated and double potentials [5]. Surrounding atrial activation can also be recorded from within the pulmonary veins and masquerades as local pulmonary vein activation. Nearby atrial activation can mask pulmonary vein myocardial activation if it is synchronous, while asynchronous atrial activation is produced by the presence of slow conduction and/or regions of block within or to the pulmonary vein and results in double potentials in bipolar recordings [6]. In the left superior pulmonary veins, a left atrial appendage potential is a nearly universal and particularly prominent contributor of far-field potentials (Fig. 7.1); in the left inferior veins, a lower-amplitude contribution from the low left atrium in the vicinity of the ostium is recorded. In the right superior pulmonary veins, potentials from the adjacent high right atrium and superior caval vein can frequently be recorded [7]. Recordings from the right inferior pulmonary veins typically show prominent ostial (left atrial) potentials.

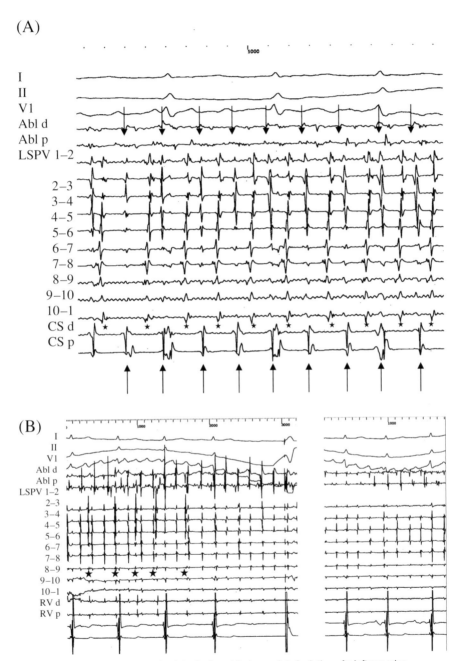

Fig. 7.1 An example of electrophysiologically guided complete isolation of a left superior pulmonary vein (LSPV) during atrial fibrillation. (A) Recordings before ablation. Two components can be recognized: the first is restricted to five bipoles and coincides with distal coronary sinus activation (arrows) representing the far field left atrial appendage potential, while the second is recorded nearly circumferentially (stars) and is the pulmonary vein myocardial potential. (B) Ablation at the inputs into the vein eliminates the second potential during ongoing RF delivery, leaving the first one unchanged as seen in the right-hand panel.

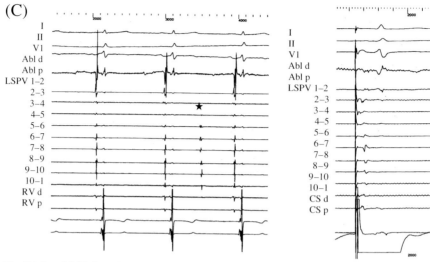

Fig. 7.1 (cont'd) (C) Complete isolation in spite of the persisting potential is verified in sinus rhythm (without further ablation to the LSPV). On the left a dissociated pulmonary vein potential is seen; on the right, the absence of a second delayed potential during distal coronary sinus pacing confirms complete isolation.

When double or multiple potentials are recorded (in sinus rhythm for the right superior pulmonary veins or during coronary sinus pacing for the left pulmonary veins) validation is relatively simple. A search is performed for clearly atrial positions in the vicinity with local activation timing matching either of the potentials recorded within the vein during at least two different forms of activation (e.g. sinus rhythm and distal coronary sinus pacing). A short or no activation delay during stimulation at threshold amplitudes from this site confirms local atrial (non-pulmonary vein) origin of that potential. On the other hand, sharp (high dV/dt or narrow duration) potentials with a long(er) activation time which exhibit a proximal-to-distal activation sequence within the vein (in sinus rhythm) are typical of pulmonary vein myocardial activation [6]; of course, the gold standard of validation is their disappearance by proximal (ostial) ablation.

The electrophysiological properties of the pulmonary vein myocardium have only recently undergone detailed evaluation. The recent introduction of preshaped circular mapping catheters has shown that activation of the pulmonary veins is asymmetrical rather than symmetrical: specific segments of the circumference are activated earlier than others [8]. This is dependent upon atrial activation and different pacing sites can be used to highlight sites of early activation. The substrate of these sites/segments of early activation remains unclear, though evidence from canine studies suggests that fiber orientation plays an important role in affecting pulmonary vein activation. Evidence obtained from catheter mapping and ablation targeting these inputs (see below) suggests that conduction block exists in part of the circumference – the result of anisotropy and fiber orientation and/or a mismatch of refractory periods or anatomical alterations such as scars or fibrous areas. The mechanism of arrhythmogenesis in pulmonary vein myocardium is not clear. Decremental conduction has been demonstrated both from the left atrium to the veins and vice versa, though the exact site of slow conduction has not been documented. Shorter refractory periods distal to the venoatrial junction combined with heterogeneity of refractoriness have been described in patients with AF [9]. Whether this reflects accentuated electrophysiological remodeling or is a more causal element in arrhythmogenesis remains to be seen. Slow and decremental conduction in the pulmonary vein myocardium and at the ostia [2, 9], coupled with heterogeneity of refractoriness (supported by the occurrence of exit block to the left atrium), renders the venoatrial junction a ripe substrate for re-entry. Evidence of electrical interconnections between left-sided pulmonary veins has recently been presented which may reflect specific anatomical variations, such as closely spaced or common ostia [10], and may contribute to the arrhythmogenic milieu in this region.

Recordings from culprit pulmonary veins during initiation of a paroxysm of AF reveal at least two distinct phases. Earliest ectopic activation typically follows sinus rhythm activation by about 200 ms and the inability to document intervening activation suggests that abnormal impulse generation is responsible. Repetitive activation in the same pattern can frequently be discerned for a few more beats at short cycle lengths (of about 200 ms), following which activation sequences become difficult or impossible to follow because of fractionation and continuous and/or changing activation. An intermediate phase with a change in intra-pulmonary vein activation without change in the surface ECG P-wave and/or intra-atrial activation is compatible with re-entry within the pulmonary vein, which may then spread or move to the venoatrial junction and involve the left atrium. Non-pulmonary foci from other great veins or the atrial myocardium may play similar roles, particularly in patients with persistent AF and atrial dilatation. This emphasizes the role of pulmonary venous myocardium as the initiator, though it is likely that the venoatrial junction and myocardium in the veins also help maintain AF. During AF, transient episodes of abrupt changes in pulmonary vein activation (with significant shortening of cycle length) have been observed which are interspersed during recognizably passive venous activation. These passages may represent episodic pulmonary vein discharge during AF, and many of the veins exhibiting this behavior have been found to be arrhythmogenic after cardioversion, in sinus rhythm, being the site of origin of ectopics or non-sustained tachycardias [11]. After isolation, a minority of pulmonary veins exhibit rapid isolated activity (cycle lengths as short as 115 ms). Detailed mapping achieved in one isolated instance has shown an origin distal to the venoatrial junction and rapid (short) vein activation times, suggesting a non-re-entrant mechanism [12]. That the majority of isolated pulmonary veins in AF patients do not show isolated tachycardias after ablation may be related to ablation interfering with the tachycardia substrate/mechanism, the need for a driving rhythm (triggered activity) and/or simply capricious discharge. Termination of sustained and even persistent AF has been observed during RF delivery; in our experience, AF termination does not correlate with the achievement of block into the adjacent vein and is frequently followed by continued ectopy generation or non-sustained runs of pulmonary vein tachycardia. These observations support a re-entrant mechanism maintaining AF coupled with a distinct initiating mechanism.

The venoatrial junction

The present technique of ablation aims to produce electrical disconnection between the left atrium and the pulmonary veins, and the level of ablation which affects the amount of myocardium isolated from the left atrium (LA) may affect success rates after catheter ablation. The desired level of ablation is considered to be the os of the pulmonary veins, but has not been precisely defined because, anatomically as well as histologically, the venoatrial junction cannot be distinguished from surrounding myocardium. Other surrogate markers have therefore been used to designate the venoatrial junction. The change in diameter from the vein to the left atrium can be used as a guideline: the site of intersection of tangents drawn from the pulmonary vein wall and from the left atrium demarcates the junction [13]. This method defines the venoatrial junction as the level of maximum change in diameter between the atrium and vein. Any imaging technique may be used to recognize this level, and though it has the advantage of simplicity and wide applicability it does not have any known functional correlates. Potentials originating from pulmonary vein myocardium are characterized by a higher dV/dt and narrower duration [6] and therefore the change in character from atrial to pulmonary vein potentials could be used to characterize the venoatrial junction. Moreover, continuous electrograms bridge the atrial and venous potentials at certain segments of the venous circumference, at sites of preferential inputs into the vein. These potentials may be considered to define the electrophysiological venoatrial junction. Though the optimum level of pulmonary vein isolation is not known, it should be proximal (on the left atrial side) to the earliest activation during ectopy or non-sustained arrhythmias so as to isolate this myocardium. In the absence of arrhythmias or with sustained AF, an arbitrary designation of the level of ablation has to be accepted. In our laboratory, we use the morphological definition of diameter change and supplement this by eliminating fractionated potentials in the vicinity. Surgical ablation results can be interpreted to suggest that the best outcomes have been achieved using procedures which isolate all the four pulmonary veins together, with a fall-off in cure rates when the pulmonary veins are isolated two by two or individually [14].

Ablation of the pulmonary veins

Pulmonary vein ablation has several distinguishing characteristics. First, this is a new target of ablation. Secondly the veins are a conduit for blood returning from the lungs; therefore, adverse reactions to ablation can have hemodynamic consequences. Thirdly, ablation is systematically performed to isolate the myocardium electrically. Furthermore – unique in the management of arrhythmias – a triggering mechanism and not the maintaining substrate is considered to be the target. In patients with frequent non-sustained arrhythmias such as isolated ectopy, runs of atrial tachycardia and short paroxysms of AF, it is possible to map and target the exact source of earliest activation, just as for any atrial tachycardia [15]. The vein of origin may be localized by documenting distal activation preceding proximal activation within it. However, the precise mapping necessary to ablate the source is complicated by the three-dimensional cylindrical anatomy of the vein and the presence of electrically active myocardium in or close to the first-order branches: they may all need to be explored to localize the source in spite of having bracketed the earliest activation within the main vein trunk. Unipolar electrograms are less useful than in the atria because of the smaller muscle mass in the pulmonary vein and frequent associated slow discontinuous conduction producing low-voltage fractionated electrograms. The probability of missing other arrhythmia sources within the arborization of the same vein trunk, however, may be as high as 35%. Nevertheless, in selected patients such focal ablation is successful in ablating the triggering mechanism and eliminating AF [2]. Follow-up data also suggest that the risk of hemodynamically significant stenosis increases with increasing distance from the venoatrial junction; accordingly, focal ablations inside the pulmonary vein seem to have a higher incidence of stenosis. This mapping-based focal technique (similar to that used for atrial tachycardias) is clearly difficult or impossible to implement in the absence of sufficiently frequent arrhythmia or in case of sustained AF. Isolation of pulmonary venous myocardium capable of participating in arrhythmogenesis (particularly if it can be performed without additional risk) is an attractive option. Isolation is facilitated by cul-de-sac activation within the veins in sinus rhythm and the fact that the myocardium within the veins serves no discernible function. All four pulmonary veins have become an anatomical designated target because of evidence that initiating ectopy originates from multiple pulmonary veins. Circumferential mapping has shown that segments of the ostial circumference are activated earlier than the rest and can be considered as inputs, allowing left atrial myocardial activation to enter pulmonary vein myocardium [8]. When ablation is directed at these sites of earliest activation, local pulmonary vein activation is either eliminated or delayed. Delayed pulmonary vein activation indicates other connections between the vein and the left atrium, which can be similarly localized and when ablation is directed to these newly manifest sites of earliest activation; typically, all pulmonary vein activation distal to the level of ablation is eliminated. A minority of pulmonary veins exhibit evidence of more than two distinct zones of venoatrial connections and in all about 50% of pulmonary veins can be disconnected by ablation limited to half or less of their circumference; naturally enough, however, this depends upon the level of ablation (lesser ablation is required more distally). In addition to the timing of local activation, the polarity of bipolar electrograms can provide vectorial information, and bracketing of a divergent vector has been used to localize inputs into the vein, much like coronary sinus recordings for a left-sided accessory AV connection [16]. The accuracy of this criterion depends upon an orthogonal orientation of the loop catheter (and bipole); moreover, secondary zones of wavefront curvature can reduce its accuracy. Unipolar electrograms can provide vectorial information and reduce the variability of bipolar electrograms, and have been used to guide segmental ablation. Unipolar pulmonary vein electrograms have a low signal-to-noise ratio and can be difficult to discern; therefore, like the bipolar polarity reversal criterion, unipolar electrograms also provide a complementary strategy that may be helpful in certain cases. Because the pulmonary veins are activated from the adjacent left atrium during sinus rhythm, isolation of the left atrium from the pulmonary veins is indicated by elimination of pulmonary vein myocardial potentials. Since there is no other alternative route of activation (from the LA to the pulmonary vein) which could mask persisting slow conduction, elimination of pulmonary vein myocardial potentials or their dissociation from sinus rhythm are clear evidence of conduction block. Dissociation also demonstrates the presence of block from the vein to the left atrium, but so-called entrance block (elimination of pulmonary vein potentials during sinus or a paced atrial rhythm at normal physiological rates) is also very reliable evidence of complete conduction block. Source–sink mismatch, indicated by the significantly larger atrial current source, suggests that atriovenous block is a highly specific marker of complete conduction block. Incomplete mapping probably underlies the cited instances of so-called unidirectional block. On the other hand, since not all potentials recorded from within the pulmonary veins are of pulmonary vein origin (see above), clear identification of pulmonary vein potentials is essential in order to avoid unnecessary ablation which could increase the risk of stenosis. Moreover, voltage criteria are not useful since potentials of non-venous origin persist in spite of complete pulmonary vein isolation [6, 7]. Pacing from the pulmonary veins has been proposed as an additional index in order to confirm complete conduction block from the pulmonary vein into the LA. The uneven coverage of pulmonary vein myocardium within the confines of the vein means that it is difficult to ensure stable and reproducible local capture at the same site before and after ablation, particularly since underlying potentials indicating electrically active myocardium disappear after successful ablation. Threshold effects also add to the confusion, since high-output capture of the neighboring left atrial appendage and the posterior right atrium/superior vena cava during bipolar pacing from the left and right superior pulmonary veins respectively [13].

Ongoing AF complicates the ablation procedure because the rapid and irregularly irregular activation pattern makes recognition of the earliest segments of activation and the separation of venous from non-venous potentials difficult (Fig. 7.1). However, when assessed with circumferential mapping, pulmonary vein activation sequences frequently show periods of consistent activation, without significant beat-to-beat variation, lasting up to a few seconds at a time. The ostial site of this pattern of earliest activation represents one input from the left atrium to the pulmonary vein and can be targeted by ablation. The varying beat-to-beat atrial activation characteristic of AF renders all the multiple inputs evident, and these different breakthroughs can be targeted appropriately as long as the loop catheter can be maintained in position. When earliest activation cannot be discerned because of marked interval variation combined with long-duration fractionated electrograms, anatomical ablation of the ostial circumference may be envisaged. The varying activation makes recognition of a change in pulmonary vein activation during AF more difficult: the elimination of multiple inputs renders vein activation more stereotypic, although irregular, while the disappearance of activation in part or all of the vein circumference is clear evidence of compromised conduction to the vein (Fig. 7.1). However, rate-dependent conduction block may falsely suggest successful isolation and therefore verification in sinus rhythm is necessary. Persisting potentials in the left pulmonary veins (particularly the left superior vein) may in fact be left atrial appendage potentials and confirmation requires an analysis during distal coronary sinus pacing after cardioversion (Fig. 7.1). Successful disconnection can routinely be achieved by following the above guidelines in the majority of pulmonary veins, even during AF, without prolonging the procedure or performing multiple cardioversions [17].

Complications of pulmonary vein ablation

Ablation within the low-pressure left atrium predisposes to stasis within long sheaths and necessitates good technique and careful purging in order to avoid thromboembolic complications, including those of air emboli. The use of heparin-supplemented constant-flow irrigation of long sheath sidearms can help prevent the occurrence of thromboembolic events. The close anatomical relationship of the left atrial appendage with the left superior pulmonary vein means that perforation of the appendage by probing catheters can occur if it is mistaken for the left superior pulmonary vein. Distally within the right superior pulmonary vein, the phrenic nerve is in relative proximity, though at present, with the emphasis on ostial or left atrial ablation, one is rarely distal enough to endanger the phrenic nerve. The focal approach can, however, result in a lesion affecting the phrenic nerve: unilateral hiccoughs during ablation should prompt cessation of radiofrequency (RF) energy delivery. During ablation of the left pulmonary vein ostia, a transient vagal-type response with prolongation of AV conduction, culminating in block and a drop in blood pressure, can be seen during RF energy delivery. Typically accompanied by intense pain, it may be reproducible. Atropine and fluid administration accompanied by analgesics, reduction in power output or a change in the ablation site usually suffice as management measures. The tissue response to RF delivered in the pulmonary veins can encroach on luminal integrity, with hemodynamic consequences. Segmental or unilateral pulmonary edema and even pulmonary venous infarction have been described as a result of severe pulmonary vein stenosis or occlusion – usually of more than one vein [18]. It is well known that heat-fixing the coronary arteries produces an unacceptably high incidence of stenosis (restenosis, in fact), and though the venous structure is clearly distinct, experimental studies support the supposition that RF energy-generated tissue heating is responsible for pulmonary vein stenosis [19]. Stenosis appears acutely, even immediately and during RF delivery (during intracardiac echo monitoring), and does not respond to smooth muscle relaxants. Serial angiographic follow-up suggests that mild to moderate stenosis (up to 50% stenosis) frequently improves or disappears over a period of days. Such narrowing and subsequent improvement may reflect the result of edema and inflammation, more severe stenosis reflecting the effect of greater and irreversible tissue heating on vessel wall proteins, a heat-shrink-like effect. It is not clear whether intermediate-term or long-term progression of pulmonary vein stenosis does occur, but there is clearly a need for continued surveillance and follow-up. In accordance with the above proposition, higher RF power and more extensive ablation seem to favor stenosis. Distal ablation also appears to increase the risk of stenosis, which may be related to differences in the composition of the vein wall and/or the smaller baseline lumen diameter. In our experience, 1.5% of the last 307 patients who underwent ablation of all four pulmonary veins developed pulmonary vein stenosis (defined as a diameter narrowing in excess of 50%). Two patients required balloon dilatation, including stent implantation in one. In the event of pulmonary vein narrowing being recognized during or immediately after ablation, intravenous corticosteroid therapy (a bolus of 1–2 mg/kg and then orally for a week) may help in the resolution of inflammatory changes. Diameter narrowing of more than 50% and a mean gradient of more than 5 mmHg can be considered significant; however, the presence of symptoms such as effort dyspnea or symptoms at rest or the documentation of pulmonary hypertension should prompt consideration of relieving the stenosis. Balloon dilatation can provide some relief, but restenosis is very likely; moreover, it is not clear whether stent implantation provides any additional benefit. Surgical reimplantation of the pulmonary veins may have to be considered in the event of restenosis or complete occlusion.

The electrophysiological consequence of pulmonary vein isolation is the creation of large enough zones of unexcitable tissue (ablated ostia) which could then serve as central obstacles for re-entrant arrhythmias. It follows, therefore, that larger obstacles could favor more stable re-entry by providing a longer conduction time around it; however, zones of slow conduction may stabilize even small re-entrant circuits. The elimination of fractionated potentials at vein ostia and the isolation of triggering sources may reduce the incidence of this complication.

Outcome of pulmonary vein ablation

At present the outcome of catheter isolation of the pulmonary veins is better for paroxysmal than for persistent AF patients. Approximately 75% of patients with paroxysmal AF can be rendered free of AF by isolation of all four pulmonary veins. A single-center experience of anatomical encircling of the four ostia guided by electroanatomical mapping has demonstrated even higher success rates, and in a relatively large cohort of patients which includes patients with persistent fibrillation as well [20]. Surgical efforts to minimize the long and complicated Maze procedure have also provided pointers to the importance of the posterior left atrium and the region around the ostia of the pulmonary veins: highest success rates are seen when the four pulmonary veins are isolated *en bloc* by surgical incision. Intraoperative RF ablation of the left atrium aimed at creating wide zones of block from one ostium to the other and down to the mitral annulus has also achieved good results – though AF-free rates were higher in patients with smaller atria than in patients with mitral valve disease and large atria.

Residual arrhythmias occurring after successful isolation of all the pulmonary veins suggest the presence of other triggers outside the ablated zone and, if fibrillation is sustained, the presence of a maintaining substrate as well. Non-sustained arrhythmias provide the opportunity to map and track down their source. With frequent arrhythmias as well as sufficient catheters in relevant locations, locating the source of these arrhythmias (earliest site of activation) is straightforward. At least one or two catheters in the left atrium should be coupled with others in the right atrium and the coronary sinus. When combined with insights obtained from analysis of the ectopic P wave on the surface ECG, a roving catheter may be able to concentrate mapping close to the presumed sight of origin. Since the ectopic P wave, by virtue of its short coupling interval, is concealed by the superimposed T wave of the preceding QRS, subtraction using a template QRS effectively unmasks the morphology of the ectopic, thus permitting a surprisingly accurate analysis of the site of origin [22]. However, the precise choice of an ablation site needs appropriate endocardial mapping – typically with a roving ablation catheter. A multielectrode catheter array, such as a basket catheter, allows rapid localization of the region of origin, but rove mapping is still required to decide the exact ablation site. In addition, the basket catheter may be difficult to deploy and may impede manipulation of the rove catheter. Some of the same considerations also apply to non-contact mapping performed with a balloon multielectrode array, and any additional advantages are difficult to demonstrate. The results of mapping have shown that the great majority of residual mappable triggers – non-sustained tachycardias or ectopics – originate from the posterior left atrium in the vicinity of the pulmonary veins. Many (but not all) may originate from the border of the ablated zone, as indicated by their physical proximity as well as low-amplitude fractionated electrograms at the site of successful ablation. Too distal pulmonary vein isolation may in fact be responsible by sparing (arrhythmogenic) pulmonary venous myocardium proximal to the level of ablation; alternatively, ablation border zone injury may be responsible for arrhythmias. Other sites of origin include right atrial sites and great veins such as the superior vena cava and the coronary sinus. The ligament of Marshall is the vestigial remnant of the vein of Marshall, which is derived from the left common cardinal vein. Though atretic in most individuals, it may persist as a left-sided superior vena cava and, like the right-sided superior vena cava, it may be the seat of triggering arrhythmias. These great thoracic veins possess a sheath of striated myocardium continuous with or connected to the adjacent atrium and can therefore be isolated in sinus rhythm in the same way as the pulmonary veins. The proximity of the right phrenic nerve to the (right-sided) superior vena renders it vulnerable to injury by RF energy, putting in doubt a strategy of systematic isolation in the absence of arrhythmias [23]. The vein of Marshall, in spite of being mostly atretic, possesses a core of striated myocardium and may be arrhythmogenic by virtue of connecting to the coronary sinus musculature as well as to the left atrium. Cannulation of this vestigial structure has proved to be difficult and associated with dissections or perforation [24]. It is unclear whether cannulation and/or epicardial ablation are really necessary. The arrhythmogenicity of this structure has not been shown to reach the level of prevalence of the pulmonary veins and specific anatomical targeting of this structure has not improved success rates.

There are legitimate concerns about the optimum extent of ablation, the operator-dependence of results, and long procedure times. In order to circumvent some of these issues, various innovations are being assessed. These options are mostly based on the cylindrical anatomy of the veins. A balloon or equivalent circumferential ablation device is conceptually simple yet complex in practice [21]. Present insight suggests that a proximal–ostial position is ideal and therefore a longitudinally asymmetrical cone-shaped balloon may be preferable. A balloon filled with fluid/radio-opaque contrast medium is heavy, difficult to manipulate and stabilized against the direction of blood flow. Aside from these mechanical issues, different power sources are being debated. Ultrasound, microwave, conductive thermal heating and cryoablation are all being tried with the avowed intention of improving on the results of RF energy. In view of the extensive experience with RF and its good safety record, these competitive ablative energy sources may have a long way to go, though the perceived non-stenosing nature of cryoenergy makes it a strong contender.

Left atrial linear ablation

Linear left atrial ablation is closest to surgical efforts and has been tried before pulmonary vein isolation. However, ablation catheters are better suited to point-by-point rather than atriotomy-like lesions, and have therefore been used to create a series of lesions which, if contiguous and transmural, coalesce to result in an atriotomy-like linear lesion. A close analogy would be an attempt to cut a sheet of paper with a pin that can only create little pin holes. One would have to be very precise and painstaking in order to line up sufficient holes close together so that the paper falls apart. A conventional ablation catheter is the pin in question and this analogy summarizes the difficulty encountered in producing complete linear ablation lesions. Various strategies have been used in order to render this painstaking task a little easier. One relies on long sheaths providing a 'railroad' for repeated traverses – drags – of the catheter tip over the endocardium, and another uses some form of catheter tip tracking in order to log each lesion delivery in space to try to ensure serial lesion proximity and contiguity. Both techniques have their problems. The drag technique tends to reproducibly leave gaps in the lesion line at sites of topographic irregularity and is difficult if not impossible to adapt to anatomical variation, while trying to ensure continuity of point lesions is both painstaking and difficult in the beating heart, even with sophisticated forms of catheter tip tracking. Enlarging the size of each point lesion facilitates the creation of a complete line, and both large-tip catheter electrodes (8 mm) and irrigated-tip catheters have been used to accomplish this.

The electrophysiological rationale and the premise for constructing complete linear lesions are not completely clear. The critical mass hypothesis, which postulates that a certain myocardial mass is necessary to sustain fibrillation, is often invoked to explain the efficacy of surgical procedures like Maze surgery, though, given the right conditions (slow conduction and short refractory periods), fibrillation can be sustained even in small pieces of myocardium such as the mouse heart. The Maze surgical scheme was actually conceived in a canine model with the intention of eliminating all macro-re-entrant circuits around existing anatomical barriers, such as the ostia of great veins and the AV valves. Of note, this would not eliminate functional re-entrant circuits or fixed circuits around other regions of block, which could act as mother waves and perpetuate fibrillation. Data from patients successfully treated with either Maze (or similar) surgery or catheter-based linear ablation are limited and therefore the exact mechanism whereby these procedures eliminate AF is unclear. The available data indicate that linear lesions prolong atrial activation times by forcing detours and may therefore reduce the spatiotemporal freedom of multiwavelet re-entry or wandering rotors. They may even slow conduction velocity, exclude tissue with short refractory periods, eliminate pivot points or widen the excitable gap. Anecdotal data suggest that incomplete linear lesions are associated with the recurrence of arrhythmia – more often than not, these arrhythmias are organized as flutter-like macro-re-entries; however, formal evidence that complete linear lesions are necessary in order to eliminate AF (as opposed to organized macro-re-entry) is lacking. In experimental models incomplete lesions are associated with a higher incidence of macro-re-entrant arrhythmias around them and therefore ablation lesions are extended from one region of anatomical block to another without intervening gaps. Moreover, lesions which result in minimal alteration of activation in sinus rhythm are preferable. However, it is unclear whether more linear lesions equal greater antiarrhythmic effect and whether one set of lesions is suitable for all types or patients with AF. Data from surgical as well as catheter ablation interventions suggest that, among the various possibilities, greater success is achieved by lesions within the left rather than the right atrium. Most interventions have therefore favored the left atrium and attempt to take advantage of the numerous (usually four) pulmonary vein ostia and their relative proximity to each other and the posterior mitral annulus. Different combinations of lesions joining these ostia to each other and eventually to the mitral annulus have been tried with the intention of minimizing the amount of excluded (isolated) myocardium. The longest lesion length is probably provided by a lesion sequentially extending from the right inferior to the right superior pulmonary vein and then to the left-sided superior and inferior pulmonary veins before culminating at the mitral annulus. These lesions, if complete, prevent the occurrence of re-entry around isolated ostia, ipsilateral ostia and even around all four together (which in effect is the same as re-entry around the mitral valve annulus). In practice, ostial isolation of ipsilateral pulmonary veins frequently results in coalescent lesions, which does away with the necessity of joining ipsilateral ostia by additional lesions. Evidently, this is easier if the ostia are closely spaced. The corollary is that conducting gaps would persist at the level of the pulmonary veins if pulmonary isolation is not performed.

Swartz and colleagues were the first to attempt to perform linear lesions within the left atrium [25]. Using a dual coaxial sheath system, they performed extensive ablation lesions across the roof, the lateral wall and the anterior left atrium. In a relatively small group of patients in persistent AF, stable restoration of sinus rhythm was achieved in about 80%, including even patients with dilated left atria. However, significant side-effects, including mortality, were reported and procedure times were prohibitively long, though the absence of a complete publication has left many of the details unclear. Attempts at linear ablation in the right atrium achieved poor efficacy even after extensive systematic ablation [26] and therefore led to ablation within the left atrium. In one series, lesions were delivered so as to bridge the two superior pulmonary veins, the ipsilateral inferior vein ostia and to connect them to the posterior mitral annulus. Other lesions were also delivered from the right superior pulmonary vein ostia to the mitral annulus. Many of these patients developed persistent or incessant left atrial macro-re-entry, though the rates of successful elimination of AF were significantly higher than with right atrial ablation. However, procedures were long and accompanied by not insignificant morbidity [27]. No single lesion pattern appeared essential for the successful elimination of AF, though this conclusion is limited by the inability to consistently achieve complete lesions. In this context, the recognition of the initiating role of pulmonary venous myocardium provided another target much more conducive to point-by-point catheter ablation. However, with increasing experience and the transition from focal to segmental ablation and isolation as an endpoint, success rates with pulmonary vein isolation have plateaued – at about 80% in patients with paroxysmal AF, approximately 30% of patients requiring re-ablation in the first year, but substantially lower in patients with persistent AF, atrial dilatation and/or valvular heart disease. By altering the atrial sustenance substrate, linear ablation may improve results in this segment of patients and also reduce the relatively high incidence of recurrence and re-ablation after pulmonary vein isolation in patients with paroxysmal AF. In a recent series from the Hôpital Haut-Lévêque in Bordeaux (PJ, MH),

212 patients with drug-refractory paroxysmal or persistent AF systematically underwent linear left atrial ablation after isolating all the pulmonary veins. Ablation was performed with an irrigated tip catheter by delivering point-by-point lesions from the left pulmonary vein ostia down to the mitral annulus and supplemented when necessary by lesions between both superior vein ostia. A long preformed sheath was used to stabilize the catheter and improve contact. RF powers of up to 55 watts were delivered endocardially (and at lower powers within the coronary sinus if required). Local electrogram criteria and differential pacing were used to evaluate complete block. The results show that complete linear block between the left pulmonary vein ostia and the mitral annulus can be achieved in up to 94% of patients but requires epicardial (within the coronary sinus) RF delivery in most patients. Though the antiarrhythmic drug-free success rate is 86% in patients with paroxysmal AF, only 60% of patients with persistent AF remained arrhythmia-free without antiarrhythmic drug treatment. Additional ablation strategies in this patient group may therefore be needed; whether these should be more linear lesions or more strategically placed lesions is unclear. In the above series, persistent or incessant left atrial macro-re-entry was more common in the patients with persistent AF. As pointed out earlier, complete linear lesions can prevent the development of macro-re-entry and it is therefore important to evaluate conduction across the linear lesions and eliminate residual gaps. Using the principles exemplified by lesions across the cavotricuspid isthmus, local electrogram criteria (double potentials across the length of the line) coupled with differential pacing from a multielectrode catheter within the conveniently nearby coronary sinus (comparing activation times across the line during proximal and distal coronary sinus pacing for confirmation) provide effective analysis of this short linear lesion (Fig. 7.2). Multi-electrode catheter mapping, such as is possible in the right atrium for typical atrial flutter, is difficult in the left atrium because of access issues and the different plane of the mitral valve. On the other hand, sequential mapping is useful, particularly when used in conjunction with an electroanatomical mapping system as it allows visualization of the complete detour around the region of block, and this with a single rove catheter. The accuracy of determining conduction block depends both on the extent of mapping and on the site of pacing. In this context, it is easy to obtain reliable pacing from the nearby coronary sinus, permitting the proper evaluation of lesions terminating at the posterior and lateral mitral annulus. On the other hand, it is more difficult to obtain a reliable and stable pacing site close to linear lesions created on the roof, though the left atrial appendage has been used as a pacing site, in which case the septal end of the lesion line is difficult to evaluate. More than one pacing site may be needed for proper evaluation. The eventual role of linear ablation will depend upon the facility with which desired complete lesions can be achieved without associated complications; in the current phase of evaluation, it may be better restricted to patients with recurrences in spite of effective pulmonary vein isolation.

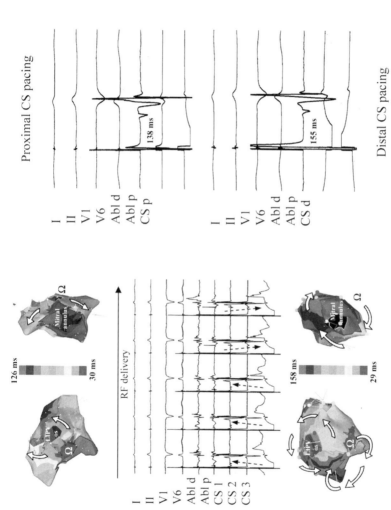

Fig. 7.2 An example of linear ablation in the left atrium between the left pulmonary vein ostia and the mitral annulus. (Top) Activation map of the LA during distal coronary sinus pacing. The arrows indicate activation wavefronts diverging around the left pulmonary vein ostia and the mitral annulus with a total left atrial activation time of 126 ms. (Middle) During RF delivery between the left inferior pulmonary vein ostium and the mitral annulus, complete conduction block is achieved, indicated by a reversal of activation in the coronary sinus and sudden activation delay in the recording from the ablation catheter. (Bottom) The left panel shows a repeat activation mapping of the LA after RF delivery, which demonstrates unidirectional activation around the left pulmonary vein ostia and the mitral annulus with a lengthening of the atrial activation time to 158 ms. The right panel shows differential pacing used to evaluate conduction across the lesion. At the top is shown the activation time across the lesion (138 ms) during pacing from the proximal coronary sinus (away from the lesion). Below it, the activation time across the lesion is shown to increase to 155 ms during pacing from the distal coronary sinus (closer to the lesion), indicating complete conduction block.

References

1 Cox JL, Scheussler RB, D'Agostino HJ *et al.* The surgical treatment of atrial fibrillation. III. Development of a definitive surgical procedure. *J Thorac Cardiovasc Surg* 1991; **101**: 569–83.

2 Haissaguerre M, Jais P, Shah DC *et al.* Spontaneous initiation of atrial fibrillation by ectopic beats originating in the pulmonary veins. *N Engl J Med* 1998; **339**: 659–66.

3 Ho SY, Cabrera JA, Tran VH *et al.* Architecture of the pulmonary veins: relevance to radiofrequency ablation. *Heart* 2001: **86**: 265–70.

4 Webb S, Brown NA, Wessels A, Anderson RH. Development of the murine pulmonary vein and its relationship to the embryonic venous sinus. *Anat Rec* 1998; **250**: 325–34.

5 Hocini M, Ho SY, Kawara T *et al.* Electrical conduction in canine pulmonary veins. Electrophysiological and anatomic correlation. *Circulation* 2002; **105**: 2442–8.

6 Shah DC, Haissaguerre M, Jais P *et al.* Left atrial appendage activity masquerading as pulmonary vein activity. *Circulation* 2002; **105**: 2821–5.

7 Shah DC, Jais P, Haissaguerre M *et al.* Analysis of right superior pulmonary vein electrograms by 3D biatrial activation mapping [abstract]. *Pacing Clin Electrophysiol* 2002; **24**: 377.

8 Haissaguerre M, Shah DC, Jais P *et al.* Electrophysiological breakthroughs from the left atrium to the pulmonary veins. *Circulation* 2000; **102**: 2463–5.

9 Jais P, Hocini M, Macle L *et al.* Distinctive electrophysiological properties of pulmonary veins in patients with atrial fibrillation. *Circulation* 2002; **106**: 2479–85

10 Takahashi A, Iesaka Y, Takahashi Y *et al.* Electrical connections between pulmonary veins: implication for ostial ablation of pulmonary veins in patients with paroxysmal atrial fibrillation. *Circulation* 2002; **105**: 2998–3003.

11 O'Donnell D, Furniss SS, Bourke JP. Paroxysmal cycle length shortening in the pulmonary veins during atrial fibrillation correlates with arrhythmogenic triggering foci in sinus rhythm. *J Cardiovasc Electrophysiol* 2002; **13**: 124–8.

12 Shah DC, Haissaguerre M, Jais P. Toward a mechanism-based understanding of atrial fibrillation. *J Cardiovasc Electrophysiol* 2001; **12**: 600–1.

13 Shah DC, Haïssaguerre M, Jaïs P *et al.* Curative catheter ablation of paroxysmal atrial fibrillation in 200 patients: strategy for presentations ranging from sustained atrial fibrillation to no arrhythmias. *PACE* 2001; **24**: 1541–58.

14 Sueda T, Nagata H, Orihashi K *et al.* Efficacy of a simple left atrial procedure for chronic atrial fibrillation in mitral valve operations. *Ann Thorac Surg* 1997; **63**: 1070–5.

15 Jaïs P, Haïssaguerre M, Shah DC *et al.* A focal source of atrial fibrillation treated by discrete radiofrequency ablation. *Circulation* 1997; **95**: 572–6.

16 Yamane T, Shah DC, Jais P *et al.* Electrogram polarity reversal as an additional indicator of breakthroughs from the left atrium to the pulmonary veins. *J Am Coll Cardiol* 2002; **39**: 1337–44.

17 Macle L, Jais P, Shah DC *et al.* Electrical disconnection of pulmonary veins during ongoing atrial fibrillation [abstract]. *Pacing Clin Electrophysiol* 2002; **24**: 456.

18 Robbins IM, Covin EV, Doyle TP *et al.* Pulmonary vein stenosis after catheter ablation of atrial fibrillation. *Circulation* 1998; **98**: 1769–75.

19 Taylor GW, Kay N, Zheng X, Bishop S, Ideker R. Pathological effects of radiofrequency energy applications in the pulmonary veins in dogs. *Circulation* 2000; **101**: 1736–42.

20 Pappone C, Oreto G, Rosanio S *et al.* Atrial electroanatomic remodeling after circumferential radiofrequency pulmonary vein ablation. Efficacy of an anatomic approach in a large cohort of patients with atrial fibrillation. *Circulation* 2001; **104**: 2539–44.

21 Natale A, Pisano E, Shewchik J *et al*. First human experience with pulmonary vein isolation using a through the balloon circumferential ultrasound ablation system for recurrent atrial fibrillation. *Circulation* 2000; **102**: 1879–82.

22 Choi KJ, Shah DC, Jais P *et al*. QRST subtraction combined with a pacemap catalogue for the prediction of ectopy source by surface electrocardiogram in patients with paroxysmal atrial fibrillation. *J Am Coll Cardiol* 2002; **40**: 2013–21.

23 Goya M, Ouyang F, Ernst S *et al*. Electroanatomic mapping and catheter ablation of breakthroughs from the right atrium to the superior vena cava in patients with atrial fibrillation. *Circulation* 2002; **106**: 1317–20.

24 Hwang C, Wu TJ, Doshi RN, Peter CT, Chen PS. Vein of Marshall cannulation for the analysis of electrical activity in patients with focal atrial fibrillation. *Circulation* 2000; **101**: 1503–5.

25 Swartz JF, Pellersels G, Silvers J *et al*. A catheter-based curative approach to atrial fibrillation in humans. *Circulation* 1994; **90**: I-335.

26 Ernst S, Schluter M, Ouyang F *et al*. Modification of the substrate for maintenance of idiopathic human atrial fibrillation: efficacy of radiofrequency ablation using nonfluoroscopic catheter guidance. *Circulation* 1999; **100**: 2085–92.

27 Jais P, Shah DC, Haissaguerre M *et al*. Efficacy and safety of septal and left atrial linear ablation for atrial fibrillation. *Am J Cardiol* 1999; **84**: 139R–146R.

CHAPTER 8

Implantable Device Therapy

Douglas A. Hettrick

Atrial tachyarrhythmias (AT), including atrial fibrillation (AF), affect over 2.2 million patients in the USA. This number may be underestimated due to asymptomatic paroxysmal AT [1]. The lifetime risk of developing AT is 25% after age 40 [2]. At present, pharmacological agents remain the primary method of disease management. However, drug therapy for rate and rhythm control in patients with chronic AT is often unsatisfactory. Recently, prevention of AT by atrial ablation has gained widespread application. Progress in this area is reviewed in detail in other chapters, but relevant to this chapter is the emerging reality that ablation is limited by issues of safety and efficacy [3]. Suffice it to say it is not a magic wand.

Device therapies for management of AT have been available for some time. The first generation of clinical devices was capable of electrically cardioverting AT with high-energy shock therapy using detection algorithms that are considered relatively primitive by today's standards [4]. Devices to terminate atrial flutter using high-frequency antitachycardia pacing have also been developed [5]. These devices have enjoyed modest clinical acceptance. For example, atrial antitachycardia pacing has been a viable therapy for patients with atrial flutter secondary to congenital heart defects [6]. Recently, a number of more sophisticated devices have been developed that combine the functions of pacemakers and implantable defibrillators with AT prevention, detection and termination capabilities. These devices have undergone fairly rigorous clinical testing for safety and efficacy. This chapter will focus on several aspects of device-based AT therapy.

Ablate and pace

Pharmacological ventricular rate control during AT can be arduous, in that it may require multiple attempts to achieve patient compliance and drug or dosage adjustment. Even with much effort, optimal rate control is frequently not achieved [7, 8]. Intolerance of optimized therapy is common, particularly among the elderly. As is discussed in detail in another chapter, atrioventricular (AV) nodal ablation with pacemaker implantation (ablate and pace) is an effective option in highly symptomatic AT patients failing pharmacological rhythm or rate control. These patients often progress to permanent AF, especially if other rhythm-controlling drugs are withdrawn [8, 9]. In selected patients (generally centering on high ventricular rate during AT), ablate and pace usually results in symptomatic improvement and can also lead to reduction in heart failure burden [10, 11]. The mechanism for the latter may be regression of the element of tachycardia-induced cardiomyopathy, which appears to be present in many AT patients with other cardiomyopathy [11]. Since AT persists in patients undergoing ablate and pace therapy, anticoagulation must be continued [12]. Another potential disadvantage of ablate and pace is that patients become pacemaker-dependent. This implies potentially high percentages of ventricular pacing, presumably from the right ventricular (RV) apex. Recent evidence indicates that RV apical pacing may lead to left ventricular dysfunction via dyssynchrony and subsequent chamber remodeling [13]. Given this, it was hypothesized that biventricular (BiV) pacing may be an alternative to RV apical pacing in patients receiving ablate and pace therapy. The recent PAVE trial was a prospective, randomized study that evaluated BiV pacing after AV nodal ablation in patients with permanent AF [14]. Patients underwent AV nodal ablation and were randomized to either BiV ($n = 146$) or RV pacing ($n = 106$). The results showed that BiV pacing improved functional capacity over RV pacing. Patients with systolic dysfunction (ejection fraction <45% or NYHA class II/III) reported greater benefit from BiV pacing, with significant improvement over RV pacing in 6-minute walk distance and quality of life assessment [14].

It has been suggested that, in addition to rate, irregularity of ventricular activation is a factor which promotes symptoms and ventricular mechanical dysfunction. Several clinical devices contain algorithms designed to promote ventricular regularity during AT. These algorithms may result in slight increases in heart rate. However, as yet none of these algorithms has been shown to diminish AT symptoms independently of rate control. In addition, in paroxysmal AT patients who are otherwise not pacemaker-dependent, these algorithms may actually be counterproductive because they force ventricular pacing. Recently, a novel method for combined rate and regularity control has been proposed, called 'coupled ventricular pacing'. The technique involves coupling a ventricular pacing stimulus to each sensed ventricular event during the relative refractory period (Fig. 8.1) [15]. In addition to ventricular rate

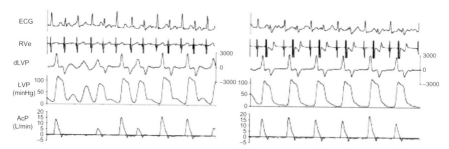

Fig. 8.1 Hemodynamic data during irregularly conducted AT (left) and during AF with coupled ventricular pacing (right). RVe = right ventricular electrogram; LVP = left ventricular pressure; AcP = aortic blood flow. (Reprinted from *American Journal of Physiology–Heart and Circulatory Physiology*, [15], used with permission from *The American Physiological Society*.)

and regularity control, the advantage of this approach is that ventricular ejection results from native rather than paced electromechanical activation. In addition, some data suggests that altered calcium handling may actually augment ventricular systolic function. At present, this technique is investigational. In addition to demonstration of incremental efficacy, issues of safety must be addressed. If these issues are resolved favorably, it is conceivable that coupled ventricular pacing may become a viable alternative to ablate and pace.

Cardioverter–defibrillator therapy

About 33% of the patients receiving an implantable cardioverter–defibrillator (ICD) for ventricular tachyarrhythmias (VT) have AT known at the time of implantation [16, 17]. One study showed that 25% had paroxysmal AT and 7% permanent AT and the yearly rate of progression was 2.6% per year for paroxysmal AT and 0.9% per year for permanent AT [16]. Therefore, up to 66% of patients with ICDs might develop AF within 10 years of implantation. Many of these patients are unaware of ongoing AT, and this may cause problems. For example, apart from the thromboembolic risk imparted by native AT, additional risk imparted by the interaction between the device and AT has been reported [18]. Patients with persistent AT at implantation also experience VT more frequently than patients in sinus rhythm and the clinical composite endpoint of death, syncope and hospitalization is three times more likely when patients are in persistent AF [19]. Dual-chamber tachycardia (VT preceded by AT) is common, suggesting that AT events actually promote VT events [20].

Dual-chamber ICDs equipped with atrial antitachycardiac pacing and automatic or patient-commanded shock (ICD-AT) have been clinically available for several years and there is substantial evidence to support their utility in managing AT. For example, Friedman and colleagues observed a significant reduction in device-quantified AT burden in patients with ICD-AT (Fig. 8.2) [21]. Similarly, Gold and colleagues reported high efficacy for AT conversion with either automatic or patient-commanded shock (87%); the median duration of successfully treated episodes was significantly shorter than for failed therapy episodes [22]. Schoels and colleagues reported a similar experience [23]. However, there are issues with ICD-AT-based arrhythmia control. Early recurrence of AT after a successful shock is one example. Schwartzman and colleagues reported the per-patient incidences of early recurrence to be 44, 61 and 70% within 1 minute, 1 hour and 1 day of a successful AT shock, respectively [24]. Swerdlow and colleagues observed that reducing the incidence of early recurrence was critical to achieving a clinically acceptable rate of sinus rhythm [25]. Interestingly, in the study mentioned above, the incidence of early recurrence fell as the duration of AT preceding the shock increased [24]. This is the inverse of what one would expect if AT was to follow a 'begetting' pattern, in which a preceding AT event duration correlates with the subsequent duration. Instead, stating that short duration (<24 hours) was unlikely

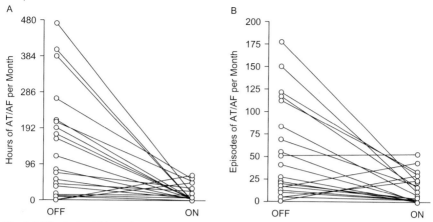

Fig. 8.2 Effect of atrial therapies on AT burden and frequency in 52 patients. (A) Comparison of AT burden in each patient between periods with atrial therapies on and off. Burden was significantly decreased during the on period. (B) Comparison of frequency of AT/AF episodes in each patient between periods with atrial therapies on and off. Non-significant reduction in frequency was observed during the on period. (Reprinted from *Circulation*, 104, Friedman *et al*. Atrial therapies reduce atrial arrhythmia burden in defibrillator recipients, 1023–8, Copyright 2001, with permission from Lippincott, Williams, and Wilkins [21].)

to exert a large effect on substrate susceptibility, the authors hypothesized that early recurrence was largely a function of trigger activity, and that trigger foci may have been suppressed by longer AT duration. This concept is now being tested in a prospective study; a positive result would introduce a technique (patience) for reducing the incidence of early recurrence. It is also likely that the addition of class I or III antiarrhythmic agents delivered in intermittent or standing oral dosage fashion reduces the incidence of early recurrence.

Another key issue with ICD-AT-based arrhythmia control is patient acceptance, particularly of ambulatory shock. Recent data suggest that the ideal candidate for ICD-AT has infrequent (perhaps monthly or longer) episodes of highly symptomatic, persistent AT and a stable, optimistic psychological profile [26]. A clear care plan and close physician oversight are also important. Anesthesia or analgesia administered at home may also improve patient acceptance. For example, a recent report demonstrated that nitrous oxide inhaled prior to shock markedly reduced pain and discomfort and ameliorated patient trepidation [27]. A similar experience has been reported with oral anxiolytic agents, particularly if the AT shock is delivered automatically rather than triggered by the patient [28, 29].

Given that the vast majority of patients with ICD have left ventricular systolic dysfunction, a key issue affecting ICD-based therapy for AT is heart failure. AT is common in heart failure, with incidence increasing as heart failure severity worsens [30–32]. From a mechanistic vantage point, it might be assumed that patients with both AT and heart failure would benefit from AT suppression, given their sensitivity to ventricular rate and regularity control and atrial systolic function. Clinical evidence supports this assumption. In terms of mortality benefit, the Framingham study is one of several which have demonstrated AT to be an independent predictor of mortality, particularly among patients with heart failure [32]. The CHF-STAT and DIAMOND-AF trials both demonstrated that AT suppression was associated with an improved mortality in AT–heart failure patients [33, 34]. However, these trials did not demonstrate that the mortality benefit was attributable to AT suppression. In addition, these and other studies have not yet made clear which elements of cardiovascular function that are altered by AT (e.g. ventricular rate, ventricular regularity, atrial contractility) are sinister. An ongoing trial will hopefully provide insight into these issues [35].

An ICD-based approach to AT control in patients with heart failure is atractive because of the VT risk innate to this population, as well as the disappointing experience with pharmacological suppression of AT due to inefficacy, intolerance and ventricular proarrhythmia. Clinical experience has been favorable. Several reports which detail the experience with the Medtronic Jewel AF™ device were based on data collected largely from patients with diminished left ventricular systolic function and class II–III heart failure [21–25]. As was typical of these reports, Friedman and colleagues demonstrated a significant AT burden reduction attributable to the device. In similar populations, Adler and colleagues and Gillis and colleagues reached similar conclusions [36, 37]. The data of Steinhaus and colleagues supported the above-mentioned concept that AT suppression promotes VT suppression [37].

Given the rapid pace of development, surging implantation rates and favorable clinical outcomes, it was inevitable that cardiac resynchronization therapy (CRT) would introduce new considerations into strategies for ICD-based AT therapy. First, given the improvement in cardiac mechanical function commonly observed after CRT, it was reasonable to hypothesize that the AT burden might recede subsequent to CRT therapy. Hügl and colleagues recently presented clinical data supporting this concept [38]. However, these data are preliminary and proof will require appropriately controlled, long-term study. Secondly, it is clear that AT can undermine CRT therapy, diminishing the percentage of ventricular beats that are paced. In early devices with dual-site ventricular sensing this also caused problems with spurious detection of VT. Thirdly, the prospect of combining CRT and AT therapies into a single device platform presents a major challenge for manufacturers. The pace and degree to which this development takes place will depend in part upon the accumulation of more data supporting the value of atrial rhythm control in this patient population.

Antitachycardia pacing

Several commercially available devices include programmable options for atrial antitachycardia pacing (AATP). As in the ventricle, both 'ramp' and 'burst' modes are available. In addition, some devices also provide 'high-frequency' (approximately 50 hertz) burst pacing. As for VT, the cycle length and duration of AT dictate the availability of AATP. Some devices have additional empirical algorithms which couple specific AATP therapies to features other than cycle length, such as atrial rate regularity. Several clinical trials have documented the ability of AATP to terminate AT without ventricular proarrhythmia in patients with and without left ventricular dysfunction [36, 39–41]. It is clear from this experience that true termination (e.g. immediately after cessation of ATP) is more likely for tachycardias with longer, more regular cycle lengths. It is also clear that cessation may be achieved by converting a uniform atrial tachyarrhythmia into atrial fibrillation, which subsequently terminates spontaneously.

That AATP has clinical utility has yet to be clearly demonstrated. The ATTEST trial randomized patients with symptomatic bradycardia and AT for which a Medtronic model 7253 had been implanted to AATP on versus off [41]. No difference in device-classified AT burden between groups was observed. However, almost 40% of the patients had no recurrence of AT throughout the follow-up period. Furthermore, patients with device therapy appeared to have more frequent short-duration episodes and fewer moderate-duration episodes, implying that AATP therapy might reduce AT episode duration. This hypothesis requires further investigation. Gillis and colleagues recently reported a reduction in device-classified AT burden in patients with higher AATP efficacy [42]. This may have indicated a higher preponderance of uniform atrial tachyarrhythmias (e.g. atrial flutter) in their cohort. In the RID-AF trial, 451 patients with ICD-AT were followed during periods of AATP on versus off. No significant difference in AT burden was observed [43]. This may have been due to the low AT burden in this population; for example, in the subgroup of patients with history of AT, a trend towards a reduction in burden was observed.

Further technological development may help to improve outcome. For example, in current devices AATP therapy is generally delivered as a single attempt early after initial AT detection, after which the device re-arms only after sinus rhythm is redetected. However, longitudinal examination of ambulatory electrocardiographic recordings reveals periods of apparently more uniform rhythm interspersed with more typical fibrillation. This raises the possibility that recurrent, 'opportunistic' AATP, possibly targeting these more uniform periods, may be more efficacious. This concept is now the focus of a prospective study. Future devices will employ digital signal processing techniques that will enable discrimination of AT based on electrogram morphology rather than solely on time elements such as rate or regularity. Israel and colleagues reported that atrial electrogram morphology was an important discriminator of AATP efficacy (Fig. 8.3) [44]. In addition to technology, accumulating experience may help to improve AATP outcome. Key elements include optimal duration of AT prior to AATP and the relative efficacies of different AATP modalities [45].

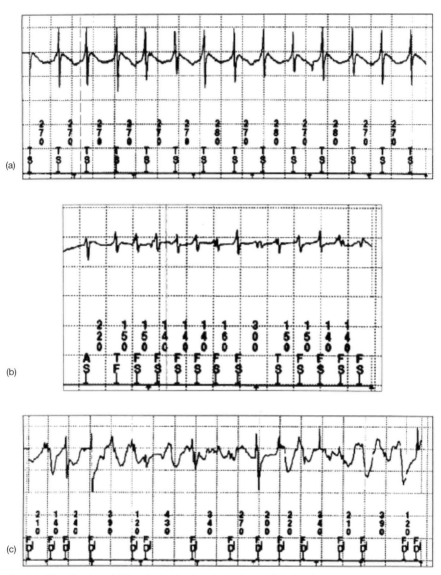

Fig. 8.3 Classification of AT on the basis of analysis of stored bipolar electrograms.
(a) Type I: highly organized AT with discrete deflections of constant morphology, an isoelectric
line between signals and a minimal cycle length >200 ms. (b) Type II: intermediate type
of organization not meeting the definition of type I or type III. (c) Type III: disorganized AT
with polymorphic deflections, no isoelectric line between signals and a minimal cycle
length, 200 ms. AS = atrial sense; FD = fibrillation detection interval; FS = fibrillation sense;
TF = tachycardia/fibrillation (overlap zone); TS = tachy sense. (Reprinted from *Journal of the
American College of Cardiology*, 38, Israel *et al*. Prevalence, characteristics and clinical
implications of regular atrial tachyarrhythmias in patients with atrial fibrillation: insights from a
study using a new implantable device, 355–6, Copyright 2001, with permission from American
College of Cardiology Foundation [44].)

Table 8.1 Algorithms for AT prevention pacing

Objective	Medtronic	Vitatron	St Jude	Guidant	Biotronic	ELA
Inhibit short–long pattern after APC	Atrial Rate Stabilization (ARS)™	Post PAC Response™				Post-Extrasystolic Pause Suppression (PEPS)™
Overdrive pace atrium	Atrial Preference Pacing (APP)™	Pace Conditioning; Rate Soothing™	AF Suppression™	Atrial Preference Pacing (APP)™	DDD+™	Sinus Rhythm Overdrive (SRO)™
Increase rate following APC		PAC Suppression™		Pro-Act™		Acceleration on PAC (APAC)™
Transiently overdrive pace atrium	Post Mode-switch overdrive pacing (PMOP)™	Recurrence Prevention™		Post-Atrial Therapy Pacing™		

Bradycardia pacing

Prevention pacing

Theoretically, atrial pacing might be expected to reduce the likelihood that AT will start. Apart from the obvious mechanism of bradycardia control, which is probably quite important in some patients because of an increased propensity for triggered activity during bradycardiac periods, pacing may serve to narrow the time or territory window by which atrial premature beats can elicit re-entry. Clinically, Andersen and colleagues demonstrated that patients who underwent right atrial demand pacing experienced a reduced incidence of AT development relative to patients who underwent ventricular-based pacing [13]. The PA trial [3] directly tested the hypothesis that atrial pacing would prevent AT occurrence in patients with symptomatic paroxysmal AT who were candidates for AV node ablation [46]. Patients were randomized to pacing with a basal rate of 70 beats/minute versus no pacing. No difference in the time to first device-classified AT was observed. Despite the neutral results of this study a host of more sophisticated algorithms for AT prevention pacing were subsequently developed (Table 8.1). At this time, among marketed brady-cardia pacing devices one or more of the following algorithms are available.

• *Constant atrial overdrive*. These algorithms are designed to achieve 100% atrial pacing. In general, these algorithms respond to sensed intrinsic (SA nodal) atrial events by transiently increasing the pacing rate (offset), maintaining the new pacing rate for a programmable number of beats (plateau), and then gradually decreasing the pacing rate (recovery).

• *Long–short prevention*. These algorithms are designed to prevent the short-long pattern of atrial events following an atrial premature beat (APB). In general, these algorithms decrease the escape interval upon sensing an APB and then gradually extend the cycle length on a beat-to-beat basis until achieving the former pacing cycle length.

• *Intermittent atrial overdrive*. These algorithms respond to APBs with constant-rate atrial or dual-chamber pacing at a fixed or variable interval above the programmed rate.

• *Early recurrence reduction*. As detailed above, early recurrence of AT is a vexing problem for device-based therapy. These algorithms seek to control atrial rate at a fixed or variable rate above the intrinsic rate for a programmable period of time after resolution of an AT episode.

Since the completion of the PA trial [3], a series of prospective randomized clinical trials have been performed in an attempt to demonstrate and quantify the utility of prevention pacing. The ADOPT-A trial was a randomized, multicenter effort enrolling approximately 400 patients with sinus node disease indicated for pacemaker and symptomatic AT [47]. The trial was performed using the Trilogy DR/Integrity AFx DR™ (St Jude Medical) and an atrial over-drive algorithm. Data from 288 patients were analyzed. Symptomatic AT events were continuously recorded with a portable patient-activated electrocardiographic monitor. Patients receiving prevention pacing had 25% fewer symptomatic AT events than those not receiving prevention pacing over a 6-month follow-up period. Symptomatic AT frequency was significantly lower in the treatment group at each follow-up visit (1, 3 and 6 months), using a covariate statistical analysis. However, the frequency of symptomatic AT events decreased progressively in both groups over time, suggesting perhaps dwindling patient compliance over the course of the follow-up. More importantly, no difference in device-recorded mode-switch frequency or duration was observed, suggesting that actual AT burden was unchanged by the therapy. In agreement with the latter, quality of life was similar between groups. A recent subgroup analysis of this trial reported that the symptomatic benefit was more pronounced in patients with less ventricular pacing [48]. The ASPECT trial was a prospective randomized 3-month crossover trial investigating the utility of a suite of algorithms containing elements of each of the four types listed above in patients with a standard indication for pacemaker and symptomatic AT [49]. In addition, atrial lead placement was also randomized to either septal or non-septal location (see below). Results from 277 of the 298 patients enrolled indicated that prevention pacing was not associated with a reduction in AT burden or improvement in quality of life. However, prevention resulted in reduced APB frequency, and symptomatic AT frequency was reduced by 47% in the subgroup of patients in whom the atrial lead was placed septally. A subsequent analysis demonstrated a reduction in device-classified AT burden in the subgroup of patients with septal lead location and high APB frequency [50]. The PIPAF trial evaluated a suite of atrial pacing prevention algorithms (Table 8.1) incorporated into the Talent™ device (ELA Medical) [51]. A total

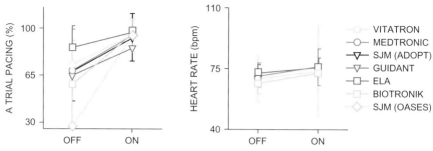

Fig. 8.4 Changes in percentage of atrial pacing (left) and heart rate (right) resulting from overdrive atrial pacing algorithms. All algorithms yielded a high percentage of pacing with modest changes in heart rate. Data are compiled from multiple reports.

of 232 patients with a standard pacemaker indication and AT were enrolled; 192 of these patients were randomized in a 6-month crossover comparing prevention on versus off. The final analysis was performed on 111 patients: no changes in mode switch duration (11.9 ± 27.7 versus 11.6 ± 26.5 days) were observed. A subsequent analysis identified a subgroup comprising patients who experienced a duration of ventricular pacing less than 70% of that recorded in the group that experienced a significant reduction in AT burden [52]. Another trial evaluated the DDD+™ overdrive algorithm in the Inos™ device (Biotronik) [53]. This trial reported 100 patients with symptomatic bradycardia and AT randomized to a 6-month crossover. The prevention algorithm resulted in increases in both heart rate and percentage atrial pacing. Despite these interventions, no change in AT (mode switch) duration or frequency could be demonstrated. Several subgroups were identified in which AT burden did decrease during periods when prevention pacing was active, including patients with sinus node dysfunction and those in whom the atrium was paced less than 80% of the time when prevention was off. No influence of the overdrive step, plateau or maximum paced rate on outcome could be demonstrated. The OASES trial was a European multicenter trial which also evaluated the St Jude Medical AF Suppression™ algorithm [54]. This trial was a crossover design evaluating either right atrial appendage (RAA) or low interatrial septal (LAS) atrial lead tip placement. A preliminary report of the outcome of this trial demonstrated significant device-recorded AF burden reduction for both lead sites, coupled with improved quality of life. Importantly, patients in this trial had a much lower incidence of atrial pacing when the prevention algorithm was turned on than in previous trials (Fig. 8.4). In that the success of prevention in this trial in reducing device-recorded burden and improving quality of life both go against preceding experience, we await a detailed publication after peer review. The PIRAT trial evaluated the efficacy of atrial overdrive pacing after AT termination [55]. Among 37 patients with symptomatic bradycardia and AT randomized to prevention on (atrial overdrive pacing at 120 beats/minute for 3 minutes following each AT episode termination) versus off for 3 months, no differences were found in AT burden.

Of note, the moment of AT recurrence frequently preceded the initiation of the prevention therapy; this is consistent with our previously reported experience with early recurrence [24]. To summarize, to date there is a lack of convincing data to support the routine use of prevention pacing for AT burden reduction [56]. However, the data do suggest that there are subsets who benefit, albeit identified retrospectively and not uniform among the studies. Pending more detailed information from preliminary reports and results from prospective studies performed on promising subsets, in view of the uniform track record for safety it seems reasonable to consider prevention pacing in patients with a conventional bradycardia pacing indication (innate or AT pharmacotherapy-induced) and symptomatic AT. At this time the data do not support considering device implantation without a standard bradycardia indication.

Promotion pacing?

As noted above, the study of Andersen and colleagues demonstrated that patients who underwent right atrial demand pacing experienced a reduced incidence of AT development relative to patients who underwent ventricular-based pacing [13]. Although this study helped to spur the development of atrial prevention pacing, it is also possible that the difference in outcomes was due to promotion of AT by ventricular pacing. A subsequent trial by the same group comparing AAIR and DDDR pacing modes in 177 patients with sinus node dysfunction also showed significantly lower AT burden among atrial pacing-based patients during long-term follow-up, associated with smaller left atrial size and better left ventricular systolic function [57]. The MOST trial compared VVI and DDD pacing modes in 2010 patients with symptomatic sinus node dysfunction [58]. The risk of AT during follow-up was slightly higher with VVI pacing. A subsequent analysis of these data demonstrated a direct association between the percentage of ventricular pacing and the incidence of AT (Fig. 8.5). The PASE trial also showed a trend towards reduced AT burden among patients with sinus node dysfunction programmed to DDDR versus VVIR modes [59]. The CTOPP trial, which randomized 1474 patients to ventricular-only pacing and 1094 patients to 'physiological pacing' [AAI(R) or DDI(R)], demonstrated significantly less AT burden in the physiological pacing group [60]. The DAVID trial found that minimization of ventricular pacing reduced the risk of combined death and heart failure hospitalization relative to a mode in which ventricular pacing was common [61].

These data support the concept that AT promotion due to pacing is a clinical reality, probably mediated by diminishment of ventricular function induced by ventricular pacing, with or without mistimed atrioventricular coupling. Common methods to counteract this, including programming of an atrial-based pacing mode or long AV delay, are often not acceptable. There has been recent progress in the development of specialized algorithms that limit the percentage of ventricular pacing compared with traditional ventricle-based pacing modes. Appropriately controlled trials are currently under way to better elucidate the value of these algorithms.

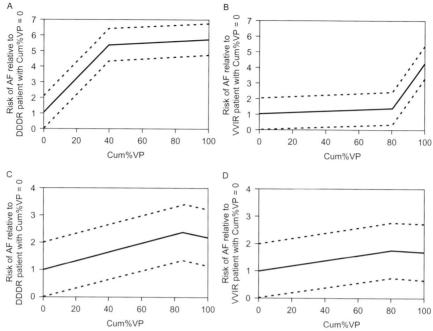

Fig. 8.5 Relation of event risk to cumulative percentage ventricular paced (Cum%VP) as estimated by Cox models with linear spline functions. Dashed lines represent 95% confidence intervals for point-by-point estimates of the hazard ratio for a 1% change in Cum%VP. (A) DDDR mode, HFH. (B) VVIR mode, HFH. (C) DDDR mode, AF. (D) VVIR mode, AF. (Reprinted from *Circulation*, 107, Sweeney *et al*. Mode selection trial investigators, 2932–7, Copyright 2003, with permission from Lippincott, Williams and Wilkins [58].)

Alternative site atrial pacing

In theory, placement of atrial pacing lead(s) at sites other than the traditional right atrial appendage may have additional efficacy in amelioration of AT burden. If true, possible mechanisms could include reduction of the time and/or territory by which an APB might provoke re-entry, or by improvement in cardiac mechanics so as to decrease atrial wall stress. Three categories of 'alternative site pacing' have thus far been tested: (i) atrial septal pacing; (ii) dual-site (free wall and septum) right atrial pacing; and (iii) biatrial pacing.

Saksena and colleagues conducted a multicenter crossover trial comparing right atrial free wall and dual-site pacing with support pacing control [62]. Patients had symptomatic bradycardia and AT. The incidence of the primary endpoint of the study, symptomatic AT recurrence, was not different between the study groups. The NIPPAF trial reported decreased time to symptomatic AT recurrence in patients with no other device indication, using a combination of atrial overdrive pacing and dual-site right atrial pacing [63]. Daubert and colleagues have espoused the benefits of biatrial pacing in patients with bradycardia, AT and inter-atrial conduction delay [64]. Bailin and colleagues reported that implantation of a single atrial lead in the high atrial septal (Bachmann's bundle) region diminished the risk of progression to persistent

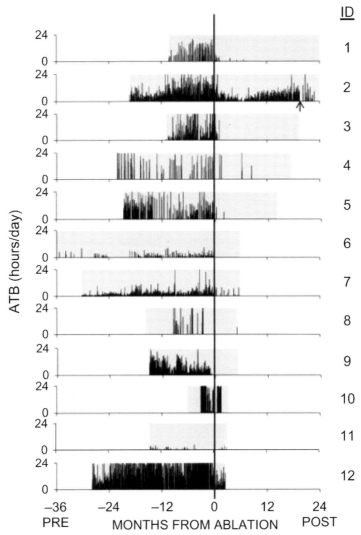

Fig. 8.6 Device-stored atrial tachyarrhythmia burden (ATB, hours/day) in 12 patients over time. Cumulative data were compiled for each patient from one or more follow-up device interrogations (AT500; Medtronic). The zero line indicates the date of the ablation procedure. ATB decreased significantly between the pre-ablation and post-ablation periods ($P < 0.01$). Gray boxes indicate duration of device implant and available follow-up burden data. One patient received an additional late-term ablation procedure (arrow). (Reprinted from *PACE*, 25, Israel CW, Analysis of mode switching algorithms in dual chamber pacemakers, 380–93, Copyright 2002, with permission from Blackwell Publishing Ltd [70].)

AF [65]. Padeletti and colleagues reported that implantation of a single atrial lead in the low septal (coronary sinus ostium) region reduced device-classified AT burden; interestingly, the addition of constant overdrive function did not improve outcome relative to simple demand pacing [66]. The ASPECT trial randomized patients with symptomatic bradycardia and AT to atrial septal (any region) or free wall right atrial pacing [67]. No significant difference in AT burden was observed.

In summary, the utility of alternative (single or multiple) site atrial pacing for control of AT remains questionable. Appropriately designed prospective studies will be necessary to further explore and define key elements, including pacing site(s), pacing algorithms and patient subsets.

Device diagnostics

An important benefit of implantable device therapy is the diagnostic information which becomes available. Sophisticated devices provide a wide range of data including AT frequency, duration, onset time/date and correlation with physical and metabolic activity. Some devices permit real-time access (office-based or remote) to diagnosis by patient or care provider. This information may be useful for vetting symptoms, assaying the risk–benefit of anticoagulation therapy, and titrating antiarrhythmic therapies. For example, in a recent report device information permitted detailed assessment of outcomes after catheter ablation (Fig. 8.6) [68]. Given the experience that symptom burden is an unreliable arbiter of electrocardiographic AT burden, an increasing number of clinical trials are using device information to define endpoints [49–54, 69].

Obviously, to realize the benefit of diagnostic information, as well as to ensure appropriate device therapy, accurate detection of AT is key [70–72]. Recent improvements in techniques and technologies for AT detection by devices has yielded increases in the positive predictive value, sensitivity and specificity of AT detection, each of which now routinely exceeds 95% [73, 74].

References

1 Feinberg WM, Blackshear JL, Laupacis A *et al*. Prevalence, age distribution and gender of patients with atrial fibrillation: analysis and implications. *Arch Intern Med* 1995; **155**: 469–73.

2 Lloyd-Jones DM, Wang TJ, Leip EP *et al*. Lifetime risk for development of atrial fibrillation: the Framingham heart study. *Circulation* 2004; **110**: 1042–6.

3 Pacifico A, Henry PD. Ablation for atrial fibrillation: are cures really achieved? *J Am Coll Cardiol* 2004; **43**: 1940–2.

4 Tse HF, Lau CP, Ayers GM. Incidence and modes of onset of early reinitiation of a trial fibrillation after successful internal cardioversion, and its prevention by intravenous sotalol. *Heart* 1999; **82**: 319–24.

5 Connelly DT, de Belder MA, Cunningham D *et al*. Long-term follow up of patients treated with a software based antitachycardia pacemaker. *Br Heart J* 1993; **69**: 250–4.

6 Stephenson EA, Casavant D, Tuzi J *et al*.; ATTEST Investigators. Efficacy of atrial anti-tachycardia pacing using the Medtronic AT500 pacemaker in patients with congenital heart disease. *Am J Cardiol* 2003; **92**: 871–6.

7 Olshansky B, Rosenfeld LE, Warner AL *et al*. The Atrial Fibrillation Follow-Up Investigation of Rhythm Management (AFFIRM) Study. *J Am Coll Cardiol* 2004; **43**: 1201–8.

8 Marshall HJ, Harris ZI, Griffith MJ, Holder RL, Gammage MD. Prospective randomized study of ablation and pacing versus medical therapy for paroxysmal atrial fibrillation: effects of pacing mode and mode-switch algorithm. *Circulation* 1999; **99**: 1587–92.

9 Gillis AM, Connolly SJ, Lacombe P *et al.* Randomized crossover comparison of DDDR versus VDD pacing after atrioventricular junction ablation for prevention of atrial fibrillation. The atrial pacing peri-ablation for paroxysmal atrial fibrillation (PA (3)) study investigators. *Circulation* 2000; **102**: 736–41.

10 Kim SG, Sompalli V, Rameneni A *et al.* Symptomatic improvement after AV nodal ablation and pacemaker implantation for refractory atrial fibrillation and atrial flutter. *Angiology* 1997; **48**: 933–8.

11 Peters KG, Kienzle MG. Severe cardiomyopathy due to chronic rapidly conducted atrial fibrillation: complete recovery after restoration of sinus rhythm. *Am J Med* 1988; **85**: 242–4.

12 Wyse DG, Waldo AL, DiMarco JP *et al.*; Atrial Fibrillation Follow-up Investigation of Rhythm Management (AFFIRM) Investigators. A comparison of rate control and rhythm control in patients with atrial fibrillation. *N Engl J Med* 2002; **347**: 1825–33.

13 Andersen HR, Nielsen JC, Thomsen PE *et al.* Long-term follow-up of patients from a randomised trial of atrial versus ventricular pacing for sick-sinus syndrome. *Lancet* 1997; **350**: 1210–16.

14 Doshi RN. Ablate and pace therapy revisited: biventricular pacing and results of the PAVE trial. In: *American College of Cardiology Annual Scientific Session*, 2004. Oral presentation; copyright © 2004 medscape. http://www.medscape.com/viewarticle/473268

15 Yamada H, Mowrey KA, Popovic ZB *et al.* Coupled pacing improves cardiac efficiency during acute atrial fibrillation with or without cardiac dysfunction. *Am J Physiol Heart Circ Physiol* 2004; **287**: H2016–22.

16 Feinberg WM, Blackshear JL, Laupacis A *et al.* Prevalence, age distribution and gender of patients with atrial fibrillation: analysis and implications. *Arch Intern Med* 1995; **155**: 469–73.

17 Best PJ, Hayes DL, Stanton MS. Potential usage of dual chamber pacing in implantable cardioverter defibrillators. *PACE* 1999; **22**: 79–85.

18 Connelly DT, de Belder MA, Cunningham D *et al.* Long-term follow up of patients treated with a software based antitachycardia pacemaker. *Br Heart J* 1993; **69**: 250–4.

19 Gronefeld GC, Mauss O, Li YG *et al.* Association between atrial fibrillation and appropriate implantable cardioverter defibrillator therapy: results from a prospective study. *J Cardiovasc Electrophysiol* 2000; **11**: 1208–14.

20 Stein KM, Euler DE, Mehra R *et al.*; Jewel AF Worldwide Investigators. Do atrial tachyarrhythmias beget ventricular tachyarrhythmias in defibrillator recipients? *J Am Coll Cardiol* 2002; **40**: 335–40.

21 Friedman PA, Dijkman B, Warman EN *et al.* Atrial therapies reduce atrial arrhythmia burden in defibrillator patients. *Circulation* 2001; **104**: 1023–8.

22 Gold MR, Sulke N, Schwartzman DS, Mehra R, Euler DE; Worldwide Jewel AF-Only Investigators. Clinical experience with a dual-chamber implantable cardioverter defibrillator to treat atrial tachyarrhythmias. *J Cardiovasc Electrophysiol* 2001; **12**: 1247–53.

23 Schoels W, Swerdlow CD, Jung W *et al.*; Worldwide Jewel AF Investigators. Worldwide clinical experience with a new dual-chamber implantable cardioverter defibrillator system. *J Cardiovasc Electrophysiol* 2001; **12**: 521–8.

24 Schwartzman D, Musley SK, Swerdlow C, Hoyt RH, Warman EN. Early recurrence of atrial fibrillation after ambulatory shock conversion. *J Am Coll Cardiol* 2002; **40**: 93–9.

25 Swerdlow CD, Schwartzman D, Hoyt R *et al.*; Worldwide Model 7250 AF-Only Investigators. Determinants of first-shock success for atrial implantable cardioverter defibrillators. *J Cardiovasc Electrophysiol* 2002; **13**: 347–54.

26 Burns JL, Sears SF, Sotile R *et al.* Do patients accept implantable atrial defibrillation therapy? Results from the Patient Atrial Shock Survey of Acceptance and Tolerance (PASSAT) Study. *J Cardiovasc Electrophysiol* 2004; **15**: 286–91.

27 Ujhelyi M, Hoyt RH, Burns K *et al.* Nitrous oxide sedation reduces discomfort caused by atrial defibrillation shocks. *Pacing Clin Electrophysiol* 2004; **27**: 485–91.

28 Mitchell AR, Spurrell PA, Gerritse BE, Sulke N. Improving the acceptability of the atrial defibrillator for the treatment of persistent atrial fibrillation: the atrial defibrillator sedation assessment study (ADSAS). *Int J Cardiol* 2004; **96**: 141–5.

29 Boodhoo L, Mitchell A, Ujhelyi M, Sulke N. Improving the acceptability of the atrial defibrillator. *Pacing Clin Electrophysiol* 2004; **27**: 910–17.

30 Middlekauff HR, Stevenson WG, Stevenson LW. Prognostic significance of atrial fibrillation in advanced heart failure a study of 390 patients. *Circulation* 1991; **84**: 40–8.

31 Carlsson J, Neuhaus KL, Charlesworth A, Skene AM, Braunwald E. Atrial fibrillation in acute myocardial infarction: Data from the TIME-II study [abstract]. *Circulation* 1999; **100**: I500.

32 Wang TJ, Larson MG, Levy D *et al.* Temporal relations of atrial fibrillation and congestive heart failure and their joint influence on mortality: the Framingham Heart Study. *Circulation* 2003; **107**: 2920–5.

33 Deedwania PC, Singh BN, Ellenbogen K *et al.* Spontaneous conversion and maintenance of sinus rhythm by amiodarone in patients with heart failure and atrial fibrillation: observations from the Veterans Affairs Congestive Heart Failure Survival Trial of Antiarrhythmic Therapy (CHF-STAT). The Department of Veterans Affairs CHF-STAT Investigators. *Circulation* 1998; **98**: 2574–9.

34 Torp-Pederson C, Moller M, Bloch-Thomsen PE *et al.* Dofetilide in patients with congestive heart failure and left ventricular dysfunction. *N Engl J Med* 1999; **341**: 857–65.

35 Roy D. Rationale for the Atrial Fibrillation and Congestive Heart Failure (AF-CHF) Trial. *Card Electrophysiol Rev* 2003; **7**: 208–10.

36 Adler SW 2nd, Wolpert C, Warman EN *et al.* Efficacy of pacing therapies for treating atrial tachyarrhythmias in patients with ventricular arrhythmias receiving a dual-chamber implantable cardioverter defibrillator. *Circulation* 2001; **104**: 887–92.

37 Steinhaus DM, Cardinal DS, Mongeon L *et al.* Internal defibrillation: pain perception of low energy shocks. *Pacing Clin Electrophysiol* 2002; **25**: 1090–3.

38 Hügl B, Mortenese P, Gasparini M *et al.* Monitoring of burden of non-persistent atrial fibrillation in the course of bi-ventricular pacing in patients with chronic heart failure [abstract]. *Circulation* 2003; **108**: IV–486.

39 Gillis AM, Unterberg-Buchwald C, Schmidinger H *et al.*; GEM III AT Worldwide Investigators. Safety and efficacy of advanced atrial pacing therapies for atrial tachyarrhythmias in patients with a new implantable dual chamber cardioverter-defibrillator. *J Am Coll Cardiol* 2002; **40**: 1653–9.

40 Israel CW, Hugl B, Unterberg C *et al.*; AT500 Verification Study Investigators. Pace-termination and pacing for prevention of atrial tachyarrhythmias: results from a multicenter study with an implantable device for atrial therapy. *J Cardiovasc Electrophysiol* 2001; **12**: 1121–8.

41 Lee MA, Weachter R, Pollak S *et al.*; ATTEST Investigators. The effect of atrial pacing therapies on atrial tachyarrhythmia burden and frequency: results of a randomized trial in patients with bradycardia and atrial tachyarrhythmias. *J Am Coll Cardiol* 2003; **41**: 1926–32.

42 Gillis AM, Koehler J, Mehra R, Hettrick DA. High atrial ATP therapy efficacy is associated with a reduction in atrial tachyarrhythmia burden [abstract]. *Heart Rhythm* 2004; **1**: S66.

43 Friedman PA, Ip JH, Jazayeri M *et al.*; RID-AF Investigators. The impact of atrial prevention and termination therapies on atrial tachyarrhythmia burden in patients receiving a dual-chamber defibrillator for ventricular arrhythmias. *J Interv Card Electrophysiol* 2004; **10**: 103–10.

44 Israel CW, Ehrlich JR, Gronefeld G *et al.* Prevalence, characteristics and clinical implications of regular atrial tachyarrhythmias in patients with atrial fibrillation: insights from a study using a new implantable device. *J Am Coll Cardiol* 2001; **38**: 355–63.

45 Hugl B, Israel CW, Unterberg C *et al.*; AT500 Verification Study Investigators. Incremental programming of atrial anti-tachycardia pacing therapies in bradycardia-indicated patients: effects on therapy efficacy and atrial tachyarrhythmia burden. *Europace* 2003; **5**: 403–9.

46 Gillis AM, Wyse DG, Connolly SJ *et al.* Atrial pacing periablation for prevention of paroxysmal atrial fibrillation. *Circulation* 1999; **99**: 2553–8.

47 Carlson MD, Ip J, Messenger J *et al.*; Atrial Dynamic Overdrive Pacing Trial (ADOPT) Investigators. A new pacemaker algorithm for the treatment of atrial fibrillation: results of the Atrial Dynamic Overdrive Pacing Trial (ADOPT). *J Am Coll Cardiol* 2003; **42**: 627–33.

48 Gold MR, Fain E, Ip J *et al.* Frequent ventricular pacing attenuates the benefit of dynamic atrial overdrive for the prevention atrial fibrillation [abstract]. *Heart Rhythm* 2004; **1**: S65.

49 Padeletti L, Purerfellner H, Adler SW *et al.*; Worldwide ASPECT Investigators. Combined efficacy of atrial septal lead placement and atrial pacing algorithms for prevention of paroxysmal atrial tachyarrhythmia. *J Cardiovasc Electrophysiol* 2003; **14**: 1189–95.

50 Harvey M, Holbrook R, Young M *et al.* Combined atrial pacing prevention algorithms reduce atrial tachyarrhythmia burden in bradycardia patients with frequent premature atrial contractions and standard atrial lead placement: ASPECT trial results [abstract]. *J Am Coll Cardiol* 2003; **41**: 88A.

51 Mabo P, Funck R, De Roy L *et al.* Impact of ventricular pacing on atrial fibrillation prevention [abstract]. *Pacing Clin Electrophysiol* 2002; **24** (II): 621.

52 Blanc JJ, Barnay J, Michaelsen J *et al.* Assessment of combined pacing algorithms in prevention of atrial fibrillation. *Pacing Clin Electrophysiol* 2002; **25** (II): 712.

53 Brachmann J, Konz KH, Allaf DA *et al.* Natural history of atrial pacing in overdrive pacing [abstract]. *Pacing Clin Electrophysiol* 2002; **25** (II): 712.

54 De Voogt W, De Vusser P, Stockman P *et al.* Atrial fibrillation suppression reduces atrial fibrillation burden on patients with paroxysmal atrial fibrillation and class 1&2 pacemaker indication-the OASES study [abstract]. *Eur Heart J* 2003; **24**: 369.

55 Israel CW, Gronefeld G, Ehrlich JR, Li YG, Hohnloser SH. Prevention of immediate reinitiation of atrial tachyarrhythmias by high-rate overdrive pacing: results from a prospective randomized trial. *J Cardiovasc Electrophysiol* 2003; **14**: 954–9.

56 Israel CW, Hohnloser SH. Pacing to prevent atrial fibrillation. *J Cardiovasc Electrophysiol* 2003; **14**: S20–6.

57 Nielsen JC, Kristensen L, Andersen HR *et al.* A randomized comparison of atrial and dual-chamber pacing in 177 consecutive patients with sick sinus syndrome: echocardiographic and clinical outcome. *J Am Coll Cardiol* 2003; **42**: 614–23.

58 Sweeney MO, Hellkamp AS, Ellenbogen KA *et al.*; Mode Selection Trial Investigators. Adverse effect of ventricular pacing on heart failure and atrial fibrillation among patients with normal baseline QRS duration in a clinical trial of pacemaker therapy for sinus node dysfunction. *Circulation* 2003; **107**: 2932–7.

59 Lamas GA, Orav EJ, Stambler BS *et al.* Quality of life and clinical outcomes in elderly patients treated with ventricular pacing as compared with dual-chamber pacing. Pacemaker Selection in the Elderly investigators. *N Engl J Med* 1998; **338**: 1097–104.

60 Connolly SJ, Kerr CR, Gent M *et al.* Effects of physiologic pacing versus ventricular pacing on the risk of stroke and death due to cardiovascular causes. Canadian Trial of Physiologic Pacing Investigators. *N Engl J Med* 2000; **342**: 1385.

61 Wilkoff B, Cook JR, Epstein AE *et al.* Dual-chamber pacing or ventricular backup pacing in patients with an implantable defibrillator; The Dual Chamber and VVI Implantable Defibrillator (DAVID) trial. *JAMA* 2002; **288**: 3115–23.

62 Saksena S, Prakash A, Ziegler P *et al.* Improved suppression of recurrent atrial fibrillation with dual-site right atrial pacing and antiarrhythmic drug therapy. *J Am Coll Cardiol* 2002; **40**: 1140–50.

63 Lau CP, Tse HF, Yu CM *et al.* Dual-site atrial pacing for atrial fibrillation in patients without bradycardia. *Am J Cardiol* 2001; **88**: 371–5.

64 D'Allonnes GR, Pavin D, Leclercq C *et al.* Long-term effects of biatrial synchronous pacing to prevent drug-refractory atrial tachyarrhythmia: a nine-year experience. *J Cardiovasc Electrophysiol* 2000; **11**: 1081–91.

65 Bailin SJ, Adler S, Giudici M. Prevention of chronic atrial fibrillation by pacing in the region of Bachmann's bundle: results of a multicenter randomized trial. *J Cardiovasc Electrophysiol* 2001; **12**: 912–17.

66 Padeletti L, Pieragnoli P, Ciapetti C *et al.* Randomized crossover comparison of right atrial appendage pacing versus interatrial septum pacing for prevention of paroxysmal atrial fibrillation in patients with sinus bradycardia. *Am Heart J* 2001; **142**: 1047–55.

67 Padeletti L, Pürerfellner H, Adler SW *et al.* Combined efficacy of atrial septal lead placement and atrial pacing algorithms for prevention of paroxysmal atrial tachyarrhythmia. *J Cardiovasc Electrophysiol* 2003; **14**(4): 1189–95.

68 Pürerfellner H, Aichinger J, Martinek M *et al.* Quantification of atrial tachyarrhythmia burden with an implantable pacemaker before and after pulmonary vein isolation. *Pacing Clin Electrophysiol* 2004; **27**: 1277–93.

69 Strickberger A, Ip J, Saksena S *et al.* Long-term sensitivity and positive predictive value of symptoms as an index of atrial tachyarrhythmia recurrence in paced patients: a report of device-based monitoring in the Natural History of Atrial Fibrillation Trial [abstract]. *J Am Coll Cardiol* 2004; **43**: 144A.

70 Israel CW. Analysis of mode switching algorithms in dual chamber pacemakers. *Pacing Clin Electrophysiol* 2002; **25**: 380–93.

71 Israel CW, Gronefeld G, Ehrlich JR, Li YG, Hohnloser SH. Prevention of immediate reinitiation of atrial tachyarrhythmias by high-rate overdrive pacing: results from a prospective randomized trial. *J Cardiovasc Electrophysiol* 2003; **14**: 954–9.

72 Friedman PA, Dijkman B, Warman E *et al.* Atrial therapies reduce atrial arrhythmia burden in defibrillator patients. *Circulation* 2001; **104**: 1023–8.

73 Pürerfellner H, Gillis AM, Holbrook R, Hettrick DA. Accuracy of atrial tachyarrhythmia detection in implantable devices with arrhythmia therapies. *Pacing Clin Electrophysiol* 2004; **27**: 983–92.

74 Passman R, Weinberg KM, Freher M *et al.* Accuracy of mode switch algorithms for detection of atrial tachyarrhythmias. *J Cardiovasc Electrophysiol* 2004; **15**: 773–7.

CHAPTER 9

Surgical Ablation Therapy I: Maze Procedure

A. Marc Gillinov, Patrick M. McCarthy

The Maze procedure is the gold standard technique for ablation-based atrial rhythm control [1–3]. In this chapter, we detail the history and practice of the Maze procedure and use it as a point of departure for further development.

Cox and colleagues designed the procedure based on experimental and clinical evidence concerning the pathophysiology of atrial fibrillation (AF) [4]. To improve results and simplify the operation, they modified the Maze procedure twice, culminating in the Cox–Maze III procedure [5]. In this procedure, incisions and cryolesions are strategically placed to interrupt the multiple re-entrant circuits that characterize AF. Right and left atrial incisions isolate the pulmonary veins, interrupt the most common re-entrant circuits, and direct the sinus impulse from the sinoatrial node to the atrioventricular node along a specified route. Multiple blind alleys off this main conduction pathway (the Maze analogy) allow electrical activation of the entire atrial myocardium. In addition, the left atrial appendage is excised. The operation restores sinus rhythm and atrioventricular synchrony, increases atrial contractility, and may eliminate the risk of atrially sourced cardioembolism. The procedure is relatively complex, requiring cardiopulmonary bypass and cardiac arrest. Although it is usually performed through a standard sternotomy, more recently we have employed a minimally invasive approach that uses a partial lower sternotomy. The operation includes multiple incisions and cryolesions in both atria (Table 9.1). The left atrial lesion set, which is the most important component of the procedure, is illustrated schematically in Fig. 9.1. With the pulmonary vein-encircling incision, the pulmonary veins and posterior left atrium are completely detached from the heart, ensuring electrical isolation of these structures. A connecting incision is carried from the pulmonary vein-encircling incision to the mitral annulus, with cryolesions created at the coronary sinus and the mitral annulus itself. These connecting lesions further segment the left atrium, preventing macro-re-entrant circuits that might cause AF or atypical left atrial flutter. The left atrial appendage is excised and a connecting incision or cryolesion links the region of the left atrial appendage to the pulmonary vein-encircling incision. If the left atrium is particularly large (e.g. exceeding 7 cm in maximum diameter), its size is reduced by resection of tissue on the dome of the left atrium and between the pulmonary veins and mitral valve. While the left atrial incisions

Incisions
Left atrium
   Pulmonary vein encircling incision
     Incision to mitral annulus
     Excision of left atrial appendage
Right atrium
   Atrial septum
   Superior vena cava to inferior vena cava
   Right atrial appendage to tricuspid annulus
   Inferior vena cava to tricuspid annulus

Cryolesions
Mitral annulus
Coronary sinus
Tricuspid annulus (2 o'clock position)
Tricuspid annulus (10 o'clock position)

Table 9.1 Components of the Cox–Maze III operation

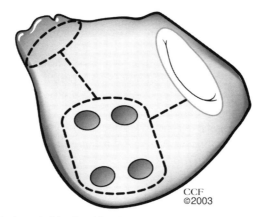

Fig. 9.1 Left atrial lesion set of the Cox–Maze III procedure. The pulmonary veins are encircled, the left atrial appendage excised, and a lesion created to the mitral annulus.

and an incision in the interatrial septum are by necessity performed with the heart arrested, the right atrial lesions may be performed on the beating heart on cardiopulmonary bypass. Right atrial incisions extend from the superior vena cava to the inferior vena cava, from the inferior vena cava to the atrioventricular groove, and from the right atrial appendage to the tricuspid annulus. In order to preserve production of atrial natriuretic factor, the right atrial appendage is no longer excised. In summary, the Cox–Maze III procedure includes seven distinct incisions and four cryolesions.

Cox and colleagues have reported the largest series of patients undergoing the Cox–Maze procedures of all types [5]. Among 346 patients, operative mortality was 2%. AF was cured in 99%, and only 2% required long-term postoperative antiarrhythmic medication. Successful ablation of AF was unaffected by the presence of mitral valve disease, left atrial size, and type of AF (paroxysmal, persistent or permanent). Transient postoperative AF was common, occurring in approximately 40% of patients. Early postoperative AF was attributed to a shortened refractory period in the perioperative period and did not diminish long-term results. Fifteen percent of patients required permanent pacemaker implantation after surgery; these were generally patients with pre-existing sinus node dysfunction; elimination of AF unmasked this underlying abnormality. Right atrial transport function was demonstrated in 98% and left atrial transport function in 93%. Late strokes were extremely rare.

Our own results mirror those of Cox and colleagues. From 1991 to 2002, 312 Cox–Maze procedures were performed at the Cleveland Clinic. The Cox–Maze I procedure was performed in 27 patients, the Cox–Maze II procedure in eight patients and the Cox–Maze III procedure in 277 patients. The indications for the procedure were broadly separated into three classes. The first group included patients with highly symptomatic lone AF who failed medical therapy, including multiple antiarrhythmic medications, and more recently, unsuccessful attempts at percutaneous AF ablation. Some of these patients had previous atrioventricular node ablation and pacemaker implantation; continued symptoms attributed to loss of atrial transport or thromboemboli prompted them to undergo the Cox–Maze procedure. The second group of patients included those with a history of thromboemboli attributed to AF. The third group of patients were those with AF (usually persistent or permanent) who required cardiac surgery for another reason, which was most commonly mitral valve disease. When AF has been present for more than a year in such patients, spontaneous return to sinus rhythm is uncommon. There were six hospital deaths and hospital mortality was 1.9%. Hospital mortality was zero for patients having isolated Cox–Maze for lone AF, 2.8% for patients having Cox–Maze/mitral valve repair, and 4.7% for patients having Cox–Maze/mitral valve replacement. Transient perioperative AF during hospitalization was common, occurring in 49% of patients. For comparison, during the same time frame, perioperative AF was observed in 39% of patients with no history of AF who had mitral valve surgery. Antiarrhythmic medications and electrical cardioversion, if necessary, were used to restore sinus or an atrially paced rhythm. AF after hospital discharge was less common and steadily decreased with time, as others have reported [3, 6]. AF occurring more than 3 months after surgery was treated by a change in medication, electrical cardioversion, or electrophysiological study with catheter ablation of the initiating source. Maze success, defined as freedom from permanent or paroxysmal AF more than 6 months after surgery, was 97.7% for Cox–Maze for lone AF, 94.4% for Cox–Maze/mitral valve repair, 95.5% for Cox–Maze/mitral valve replacement, and 100% for Cox–Maze/coronary artery bypass grafting. Overall, 3% of patients required late radiofrequency ablation for recurrent atrial fibrillation or flutter, which originated from a focus in the right atrium in most of these patients. New pacemakers were required in 10.3% (32/312) of patients early or late after surgery. Perioperative stroke occurred in one patient. Late stroke, Transient ischemic attack or other peripheral embolic event was extremely rare, occurring in only three patients (0.9%). Others have confirmed the virtual elimination of strokes by the Maze procedure [7]. This result is probably attributable to restoration of sinus rhythm and excision of the left atrial appendage, although we cannot discern the relative importance of each. These results document the safety and efficacy of the classic Cox–Maze III procedure. Other groups have reported similar outcomes in large numbers of patients [3, 8].

Recent advances in technology and the recognition of the importance of the pulmonary veins and left atrium in the pathogenesis of AF have resulted in the development of new surgical approaches to cure AF [9–13]. New operations to ablate AF employ alternative energy sources (cryothermy, microwave, radio-frequency, ultrasound, laser) and simplified left atrial lesion sets (the 'modified Maze procedure'). These operations cure AF in 70–80% of patients [9–11]. A variety of energy sources can be used to create lines of conduction block. Using either heat-based or cryo-based energy, 5-cm lines of conduction block can be created in less than 2 minutes. It requires less than 15 minutes to create a left atrial lesion set that includes pulmonary vein isolation, connecting lesions, and excision of the left atrial appendage. The rapidity and success of AF ablation using these new technologies has resulted in a much more aggressive approach to the surgical treatment of AF at our institution. Nearly all patients

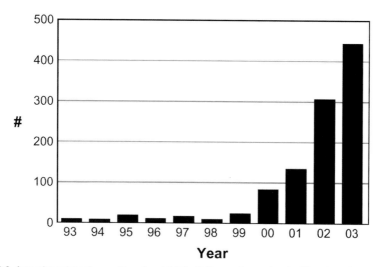

Fig. 9.2 Annual number of operations for atrial fibrillation performed at the Cleveland Clinic Foundation.

(A)

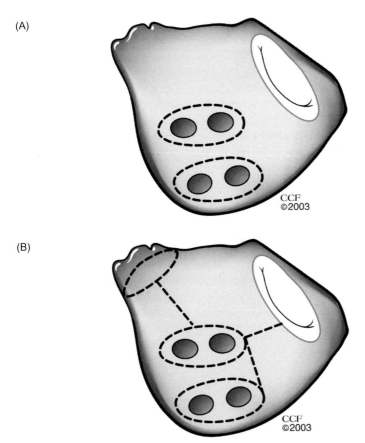

(B)

Fig. 9.3 Common lesion sets created with alternative energy sources. (A) Pulmonary vein isolation. (B) Pulmonary vein isolation with connecting lesions from the right to the left inferior pulmonary veins and from the left atrial appendage to the left pulmonary veins. The left atrial appendage is excised.

with AF who present for cardiac surgery have a surgical procedure to restore sinus rhythm. In 2003, implementation of this strategy was responsible for more than 450 surgical AF ablations at the Cleveland Clinic Foundation (Fig. 9.2). Using alternative energy sources, surgeons may create a variety of lesion sets, ranging from pulmonary vein isolation to a complete Cox–Maze III (Fig. 9.3). The ideal lesion set has not yet been identified. However, most lesion sets include pulmonary vein isolation, one or more connecting lesions, and excision or exclusion of the left atrial appendage [9]. Such lesion sets generally restore sinus rhythm in 70–80% of patients.

At the Cleveland Clinic Foundation, AF ablation strategy continues to evolve. Today, most patients having surgical ablation require concomitant cardiac surgery, most commonly mitral valve repair or replacement. For patients with persistent and permanent AF, we employ one of two approaches. In a relatively young, healthy patient undergoing straightforward surgery, we favor a classic Cox–Maze III procedure. This is the most effective time-tested curative treatment for AF, and it is relatively underused by cardiac surgeons. For elderly patients with multiple comorbid conditions or those having complex cardiac surgery, we perform pulmonary vein isolation and left atrial appendage exclusion; such patients also may receive one or more left atrial connecting lesions. Patients with paroxysmal AF are treated by pulmonary vein isolation and exclusion of the left atrial appendage. Patients with lone AF that is persistent or permanent receive a classic Cox–Maze III procedure. As noted, this approach is associated with no operative mortality and 97.7% cure of AF. Patients with lone AF that is paroxysmal receive a 'minimally invasive' procedure that includes a keyhole incision and thoracoscopically assisted pulmonary vein isolation. In the near future, it is likely that less invasive approaches for lone AF will be available. Such procedures, which will include pulmonary vein isolation and creation of left atrial lesion sets through endoscopes or small incisions, will extend the possibility of cure to large numbers of patients with AF.

References

1 Cox JL, Ad N, Palazzo T, Fitzpatrick S *et al*. Current status of the Maze procedure on the stroke rate in patients with atrial fibrillation. *J Thorac Cardiovasc Surg* 1999: **118**; 833–40.
2 McCarthy PM, Gillinov AM, Castle L, Chung M, Cosgrove DM. The Cox–Maze procedure: the Cleveland Clinic experience. *Semin Thorac Cardiovasc Surg* 2000; **12**: 25–9.
3 Schaff HV, Dearani JA, Daly RC, Orszulak TA, Danielson GK. Cox–Maze procedure for atrial fibrillation: May Clinic experience. *Semin Thorac Cardiovasc Surg* 2000; **12**: 30–7.
4 Cox JL, Schuessler RB, D'Agostino HJ Jr *et al*. The surgical treatment of atrial fibrillation: III development of a definitive surgical procedure. *J Thorac Cardiovasc Surg* 1991; **101**: 569–83.
5 Cox JL, Schuessler RB, Boineau JP. The development of the Maze procedure for the treatment of atrial fibrillation. *Semin Thorac Cardiovasc Surg* 2000; **12**: 2–14.
6 Ad N, Pirovic EA, Kim YD *et al*. Observations on the perioperative management of patients undergoing the Maze procedure. *Semin Thorac Cardiovasc Surg* 2000; **12**: 63–7.
7 Cox JL, Ad N, Palazzo T. Impact of the Maze procedure on the stroke rate in patients with atrial fibrillation. *J Thorac Cardiovasc Surg* 1999; **118**: 833–40.
8 Arcidi JM Jr, Doty DB, Millar RC. The Maze procedure: the LDS Hospital experience. *Semin Thorac Cardiovasc Surg* 2000; **12**: 38–43.
9 Gillinov AM, Blackstone EH, McCarthy PM. Atrial fibrillation: current surgical options and their assessment. *Ann Thorac Surg* 2002; **74**: 2210–17.
10 Cox JL, Ad N. New surgical and catheter-based modifications of the Maze procedure. *Semin Thorac Cardiovasc Surg* 2000; **12**: 15–19.
11 Gillinov AM, Smedira NG, Cosgrove DM. Microwave ablation of atrial fibrillation during mitral valve surgery. *Ann Thorac Surg* 2002; **74**: 1259–61.

12 Sie HT, Beukema WP, Misier AR *et al.* Radiofrequency modified Maze in patients with atrial fibrillation undergoing concomitant cardiac surgery. *J Thorac Cardiovasc Surg* 2001; **122**: 249–56.

13 Gillinov AM, McCarthy PM. Atricure bipolar radiofrequency clamp for ablation of atrial fibrillation. *Ann Thorac Surg* 2002; **74**: 2165–8.

CHAPTER 10

Surgical Ablation Therapy II: Endocardium-Based Catheter Ablation

Hauw T. Sie, Willem P. Beukema, Arif Elvan, Anand R. Ramdat Misier

Since the early 1980s, several surgical procedures have been described for the suppression of atrial fibrillation (AF). Although the Maze III procedure (see Chapter 9) has an excellent outcome in experienced hands, it is a relatively complex operation, adding to a cardioplegic interval which may already be significant due to concomitant surgery. For the past decade, an effort has been under way to achieve the Maze electrophysiological result with a simpler/ faster procedure. A key element in this development has been the replacement of the 'cut-and-sew' ablation lesion with non-incisional ablation lesions. At least in theory, these lesions achieve the same result as cut and sew but may be deployed without atriotomy, possibly in the beating heart. In this chapter, we briefly review the path of surgical development and focus on the state of the art of a 'modified' Maze procedure using catheter ablation applied to the endocardial aspect of the atrium. Included is a discussion of the various ablation energy sources which have been used for this purpose.

Left atrial isolation procedure

This procedure was developed by Williams and Cox and reported in the early 1980s [1]. Surgical isolation of the left atrium circumvents the interruption of sinus node activity, permitting sinus activation of the atrioventricular junction and ventricles. This procedure was initially developed to treat atrial tachycardias originating from the left atrium. Graffigna and associates reported results on a group of 100 patients who underwent concomitant left atrial isolation and mitral valve surgery [2]. In the early postoperative period 81% of patients were in sinus rhythm, which persisted at 2 years in 70%. The investigators concluded that the procedure is simple, does not significantly prolong cardioplegic interval, and is associated with a reasonable rate of success. However, the definition of success is based on preservation of sinus node function but neglects the left atrium, which remains in atrial tachyarrhythmia or becomes electrically quiescent after the procedure, both of which may present thromboembolic risk. Long-term anticoagulation therapy is therefore mandatory. In addition, the loss of left atrium mechanical contribution is suboptimal.

Corridor procedure

In 1985 a procedure was described by Guiraudon and his associates in which a protected 'corridor' of right atrial tissue was created to permit sinus activity to propagate to the atrioventricular node region, despite the possible presence of AF in areas outside the corridor [3, 4]. The first report from this group demonstrated success in most patients, but with a high incidence of sinus node dysfunction necessitating a permanent pacemaker. In a larger group of patients, Defauw and colleagues demonstrated success in 86% of patients, although a significant number of patients subsequently underwent an ablate and pace procedure [5, 6]. Contractile function of the left atrium was absent in all patients, regardless of its electrical rhythm; thus, continuous anticoagulation was necessary. Perioperative morbidity was significant. There were two strokes in the early postoperative period. Biatrial enlargement occurred in the majority of patients on echocardiographic follow-up.

Maze procedure

The concept of the Maze procedure was conceived in the animal laboratory based on Moe's theory of multiple wavelets [7]. After extensive animal experiments, the Maze operation was introduced into clinical practice in 1987 [8]. The procedure was subsequently modified in response to perioperative problems, such as sinus node dysfunction, resulting in its current iteration, Maze III [9, 10]. The procedure conceptualizes non-isolating electrical segmentation of the atria by multiple full-thickness atrial incisions (cut and sew), creating a labyrinth with several blind alleys in which the amount of atrial myocardium in each compartment is insufficient to sustain re-entry. The sinus impulse traverses an intact route to the atrioventricular node, eventually activating all atrial tissue (Fig. 10.1).

Initially, the Maze procedure was performed primarily in isolation; that is, without the need for concomitant cardiac surgery. Cox and colleagues reported electrophysiological success in more than 95% of these patients during a long follow-up interval [10]. This outcome was reproduced in other centers [11–13]. Although there were issues with procedural morbidity (especially sinus node dysfunction and edema), mortality was rare. Atrial mechanical function, defined by echocardiographic Doppler A wave, was demonstrable in association with postoperative electrocardiographic sinus rhythm.

Given developments in non-surgical techniques for atrial rhythm control, the Maze procedure at present has been relegated largely to patients with structural heart disease in need of concomitant cardiac surgery. Many of these patients need mitral valve surgery. In the majority of patients with AF and mitral valve disease, valve surgery alone will not eliminate the arrhythmia [14, 15]. Excellent results have been described for the Maze surgery concomitant with other cardiac surgery; long-term success rates in excess of 90% are standard [16–22]. Though effective, the procedure markedly complicates the operation,

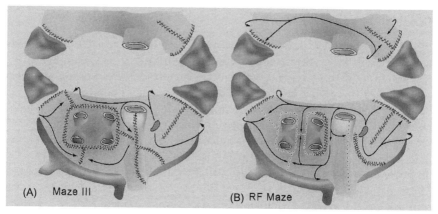

Fig. 10.1 Schematic drawing of the posterior aspect of the heart. (A) Maze III procedure. Incisions and suture lines are depicted as zigzag lines. Posterior left atrium, including all pulmonary veins orifices, is isolated. (B) Modified Maze procedure. Incisions and suture lines are depicted as zigzag lines. Radiofrequency ablation lines are shown as dotted lines. The pulmonary veins are isolated separately.

including the approach and duration, and significantly increases the risk of morbidity and mortality. Combined with the complexity of the operation, these factors have prevented widespread application of the procedure.

Modifications of the cut-and-sew Maze procedure

The efficacy of the Maze procedure drove surgical development of modifications which would render the procedure technically easier and faster. One key element in this evolution has been the replacement of cut-and-sew lesions with ablation lesions applied by catheter. When applied successfully, these lesions result in the same chronic electrical conduction block produced by incision. Various forms of energy have been used.

Radiofrequency energy (RF)

At present, this is by far the most commonly used type of energy. In clinical practice RF is delivered at approximately 500 MHz between two electrodes, the ablation (active) electrode and a distant ground electrode. The ablation electrode is mounted on a catheter which is hand-held and manipulated into target tissue contact by the surgeon. Passage of current from the active electrode to the interfaced myocardium produces molecular friction and heat, which in sufficient quantity can produce cell death. Over weeks to months, dead myocardium is replaced by a collagenous scar which is electrically inert, similar to the histological appearance of a healed incision. RF may be applied using an electrode which is irrigated with a fluid such as saline to permit more effective energy delivery. Using RF to replace cut-and-sew lesions, we performed modified Maze surgery on 122 patients (Fig. 10.1) [23, 24]. The majority of patients (89%) also underwent concomitant surgery, principally on the mitral valve. All RF lesions were applied to the endocardial surface in a still, dry heart. The additional cardioplegic interval required to perform the procedure was between 10 and 15 minutes, a marked reduction from our cut-and-sew experience. Perioperative morbidity and mortality rates were similar to those in patients not undergoing the modified Maze procedure, although we have not as yet looked at this in randomized fashion. Suppression of AF was achieved in over 70% of patients, although long-term follow-up is lacking. This experience has been reproduced by others [25, 26]. Although simpler than cut and sew, RF ablation lesions are not without their risks, including damage to non-atrial structures contiguous to the ablation site [25, 27]. In addition, there remain issues with ensuring transmurality of the lesion after the healing phase is complete. Recently, a new 'clamp' ablation catheter design has been introduced, which results in more reliably transmural lesions [28].

Cryothermal energy (cryo)

Cryo produces cell death by freezing. It has been used for years during arrhythmia surgery, including certain regions during the Maze procedure. Potential advantages of a broader use of cryo (versus RF) in modified Maze surgery include the fact that adherence of the electrode during energy delivery is associated with adherence which eliminates contact variation (which is sometimes problematic during RF application) and the diminished incidence of endocardial charring at the ablation site. Nakajima and colleagues reported a large cohort which underwent modified Maze surgery [29]. Actuarial freedom from recurrence of AF at 3 years was 97%, which was similar to their cut-and-sew Maze experience. As in reports of RF-based ablation, the cryo procedure was associated with marked diminishment in cardioplegic interval relative to cut-and-sew Maze [29]. Despite reports such as these, significant questions remain about the reliability of cryo for producing transmural atrial lesions.

Microwave energy (MW)

In clinical practice, MW is delivered at approximately 2 gigahertz through an electrode mounted on a catheter. It results in cell death by heat produced by oscillation of water molecules. Potential advantages relative to RF include larger lesion volume, diminished incidence of charring at the electrode–tissue interface, and the ability to heat through adipose tissue by convection rather than conduction (the means by which RF causes heating at a distance) [30]. Knaut and colleagues reported the outcome of an AF cohort which underwent modified Maze surgery using MW [31]. As in other reports of the non-cut-and-sew technique, Maze-attributable cardioplegia time was diminished relative to cut-and-sew Maze. At 1 year, 58% of their patients were in sinus rhythm. The advantages of the use of MW stated above, if true, may make it better suited to epicardium-based use. Maessen and colleagues reported promising efficacy in patients who underwent beating-heart epicardium-based atrial ablation using MW [32]. This approach will be discussed in detail in Chapter 11.

Laser

Laser (light amplification by stimulated emission of radiation energy) is photonic energy of a specific wavelength. Laser energy consists of a monochromatic, phase-coherent beam. The potential advantage of laser is that it can be delivered in a highly focused beam of energy of specified duration and intensity. Laser energy delivery causes volumetric heating and peak temperature below the endocardial surface, reducing charring. Endocardial application of a linear diffuser with a diode laser source has been demonstrated to produce linear transmural conduction block in the trabeculated anterior right atrial wall in a goat model [33]. Using a beam splitter, a laser balloon has been developed to project a ring of laser energy forward of the inflated balloon for the purpose of pulmonary vein isolation [34]. Vigilance and colleagues recently described their initial experience with laser atrial ablation in 6 patients [35].

Ultrasound energy

Ultrasound (US) energy is absorbed by tissue at an acoustic interface (e.g. blood–myocardium), resulting in the accumulation of heat. It has the theoretical advantages of contact independence and focusing [36]. Saliba and colleagues reported their experience with endocardium-based, beating heart ablation using a US transducer operating at 9 megahertz mounted in the center of a saline-filled balloon [36]. The balloon was inflated to occlude the ostium of a pulmonary vein. They noted that uniform and complete contact of the balloon was essential in order to produce a contiguous lesion, thus undermining one of the theoretical advantages of using US noted above.

As noted above, the efficacy of the Maze procedure has driven surgical development of modifications which would render the procedure technically easier and faster. A second key element in this evolution has been attempts to reduce the lesion burden. Nitta and colleagues reported a procedure in which cut-and-sew lesions were applied in a radial pattern emanating from the posterior left atrium [37, 38]. The lesions in this procedure are technically easier than in the Maze procedure. The authors also suggest that left atrium mechanical function is better preserved than after the Maze procedure. Efficacy rates are similar to those reported for classical Maze surgery at experienced centers [39]. A similar procedure reported by Thomas and colleagues using RF catheter lesions also conceptualized the simplification and optimization of sinus electromechanical function [40]. In a small cohort, successful AF suppression was maintained in 65% of patients at 16 months.

Experimental and clinical evidence both point to the left atrium as the seat of AF in man. One modification of the Maze procedure which has thus been explored has been to completely remove the right atrium from the lesion paradigm. Szalay and colleagues reported their experience with this procedure, comparing it with standard Maze. Albeit with small numbers, they noted no difference in clinical success of these procedures at 1 year [41]. Knaut and colleagues used MW energy to perform a similar procedure in a larger cohort [31].

This procedure has been performed with other energy sources, with varying results [42, 43]. Some have suggested that more advanced atrial disease may necessitate a biatrial approach [44].

More recently, there have been reports of attempts to further minimize the ablation lesion burden by focusing only on the posterior portion of the left atrium. As described in the foregoing chapters, the region of the left atrium contiguous to the pulmonary veins appears to be critical for AF initiation and sustenance. From a surgical standpoint, limiting the ablation target to the posterior left atrium is attractive for its technical simplicity and rapid deployment. Melo and colleagues performed intraoperative endocardium-based bilateral isolation of the pulmonary veins in patients undergoing mitral valve procedures, which was successful in restoration of sustained sinus rhythm in approximately 70% of patients [45].

Conclusion

Although the classical cut-and-sew Maze procedure is mature and quite successful in suppression of AF, surgical ablation is in a state of rapid evolution. As we have detailed, the main engines of change include techniques to replace atrial incision and minimization of the lesion burden. As yet, data do not provide clarity as to whether and which modified procedure will approach classical Maze outcomes.

References

1 Williams JM, Ungerleider RM, Lofland GK, Cox JL. Left atrial isolation. New technique for the treatment of supraventricular arrhythmias. *J Thorac Cardiovasc Surg* 1980; **80**: 373–80.

2 Graffigna A, Pagani F, Minzioni G, Salemo J, Vigano M. Left atrial isolation associated with mitral valve operations. *Ann Thorac Surg* 1992; **54**:1093–7.

3 Guiraudon GM, Campbell CS, Jones DL, McLellan DG, McDonald JL. Combined sino-atrial node atrio-ventricular isolation: a surgical alternative to His bundle ablation in patients with atrial fibrillation. *Circulation* 1985; **72** (Suppl. 3): 220.

4 Leitch JW, Klein G, Yee R, Guiraudon G. Sinus node-atrioventricular node isolation: long-term results with the 'corridor' operation for atrial fibrillation. *J Am Coll Cardiol* 1991: 15; **17**: 970–5.

5 Defauw J, Van Hemel NM, Kingma JH *et al*. The corridor operation as an alternative in the treatment of atrial fibrillation. In: Kingma JH, Van Hemel NM, Lie KI, eds. *Atrial Fibrillation, a Treatable Disease?* Dordrecht: Kluwer, 1992: 167–81.

6 Van Hemel NM, Defauw JJ, Kingma JH *et al*. Long-term results of the corridor operation for atrial fibrillation. *Br Heart J* 1994; **71**: 170–6.

7 Moe GK. On the multiple wavelet hypothesis of atrial fibrillation. *Arch Int Pharmacodyn Ther* 1962; **140**: 183–8.

8 Cox JL, Boineau JP, Schuessler RB *et al*. Successful surgical treatment of atrial fibrillation. *JAMA* 1991; **266**: 530–7.

9 Cox JL, Jaquiss RDB, Schuessler RB, Boineau JP. Modification of the maze procedure for atrial flutter and atrial fibrillation. II. Surgical technique of the maze III procedure. *J Thorac Cardiovasc Surg* 1995; **110**: 485–95.

10 Cox JL, Schuessler RB, D'Agostino HJ Jr *et al*. The surgical treatment of atrial fibrillation. (III) Development of a definitive surgical procedure. *J Thorac Cardiovasc Surg* 1991; **101**: 569–83.

11 Cox JL, Boineau JP, Schuessler RB, Kater KM, Lappas DG. Five-year experience with the maze procedure for atrial fibrillation. *Ann Thorac Surg* 1993; **56**: 814–23; discussion 823–4.

12 Jessurun ER, van Hemel NM, Defauw JA *et al*. Results of maze surgery for lone paroxysmal atrial fibrillation. *Circulation* 2000; **101**: 1559–67.

13 Lonnerholm S, Blomstrom P, Nilsson L *et al*. Effects of the maze operation on health-related quality of life in patients with atrial fibrillation. *Circulation* 2000; **101**: 2607–11.

14 Lonnerholm S, Blomstrom P, Nilsson L, Blomstrom-Lundqvist C. Atrial size and transport function after the Maze III procedure for paroxysmal atrial fibrillation. *Ann Thorac Surg* 2002; **73**: 107–11.

15 Chua LY, Schaff HV, Orszulak TA, Morris JJ. Outcome of mitral valve repair in patients with preoperative atrial fibrillation. *J Thorac Cardiovasc Surg* 1994; **107**: 408–1.

16 Jessurun ER. *Maze surgery for atrial fibrillation*. Thesis, 2001. ISBN 90-393-2861-7.

17 Hioki M, Ikeshita M, Iedokoro Y *et al*. Successful combined operation for mitral stenosis and atrial fibrillation. *Ann Thorac Surg* 1993; **55**: 776–8.

18 Kosakai Y, Kawaguchi AT, Isobe F *et al*. Cox Maze procedure for chronic atrial fibrillation associated with mitral valve disease. *J Thorac Cardiovasc Surg* 1994; **108**: 1049–55.

19 Izumoto H, Kawazoe K, Kitahara H, Kamata J. Operative results after Cox/maze procedure combined with mitral valve operation. *Ann Thorac Surg* 1998; **66**: 800–4.

20 Kim KB, Cho KR, Sohn DW, Ahn H, Rho JR. The Cox-Maze III procedure for atrial fibrillation associated with rheumatic mitral valve disease. *Ann Thorac Surg* 1999; **68**: 799–803.

21 Handa N, Schaff HV, Morris JJ, Anderson BJ, Kopecky SL, Enriquez-Sarano M. Outcome of valve repair and the Cox maze procedure for mitral regurgitation and associated atrial fibrillation. *J Thorac Cardiovasc Surg* 1999; **118**: 626–35.

22 Yuda S, Nakatani S, Kosakai Y, Yamagishi M, Miyatake K. Long-term follow-up of atrial contraction after the maze procedure in patients with mitral valve disease. *J Am Coll Cardiol* 2001; **37**: 1622–7.

23 Sie HT, Beukema WP, Ramdat Misier AR *et al*. The radiofrequency modified maze procedure. A less invasive surgical approach to atrial fibrillation during open-heart surgery. *Eur J Cardiothor Surg* 2001; **19**: 443–7.

24 Sie HT, Beukema WP, Ramdat Misier AR *et al*. Radiofrequency modified maze in patients with atrial fibrillation undergoing concomitant cardiac surgery. *J Thorac Cardiovasc Surg* 2001; **122**: 249–56.

25 Khargi K, Deneke T, Haardt H *et al*. Saline-irrigated cooled-tip radiofrequency ablation is an effective technique to perform the maze procedure. *Ann Thorac Surg* 2001; **72**: S1090–5.

26 Guden M, Akpinar B, Sanisoglu I, Sagbas E, Bayindir O. Intraoperative saline-irrigated radiofrequency modified Maze procedure for atrial fibrillation. *Ann Thorac Surg* 2002; **74**: S1301–6.

27 Gillinov M, Petterson G, Rice TW. Esophageal injury during radiofrequency ablation of atrial fibrillation. *J Thorac Cardiovasc Surg* 2001; **122**: 1239–40.

28 Bonanomi G, Schwartzman D, Francischelli D, Zenati M. A new device for beating heart bipolar radiofrequency atrial ablation. *J Thorac Cardiovasc Surg* 2003; **126**: 1859–66.

29 Nakajima H, Kobayashi J, Bando K *et al*. The effect of cryo-maze procedure on early and intermediate term outcome in mitral valve disease: case matched study. *Circulation* 2002; **106** (12 Suppl. 1): I46–I50.

30 Williams MR, Knaut M, Berube D, Oz MC. Application of microwave energy in cardiac tissue ablation: from in vitro analyses to clinical use. *Ann Thorac Surg* 2002; **74**: 1500–5.

31 Knaut M, Tugtekin SM, Spitzer S, Gulielmos V. Combined atrial fibrillation and mitral valve surgery using microwave technology. *Semin Thorac Cardiovasc Surg* 2002; **14**: 226–31.

32 Maessen JG, Nijs JF, Smeets JL, Vainer J, Mochtar B. Beating-heart surgical treatment of atrial fibrillation with microwave ablation. *Ann Thorac Surg* 2002; **74**: S1307–11.

33 Keane D, Ruskin JN. Linear atrial ablation with a diode laser and fiberoptic catheter. *Circulation* 1999; **100**: e59–60.

34 Lemery R, Veinot JP, Tang AS *et al*. Fiberoptic balloon catheter ablation of pulmonary vein ostia in pigs using photonic energy delivery with diode laser. *Pacing Clin Electrophysiol* 2002; **25**: 32–6.

35 Vigilance DW, Williams M, Garrido M *et al*. Atrial fibrillation surgery using linear laser technology. *Heart Surg Forum* 2003; **6**: 121.

36 Saliba W, Wilber D, Packer D *et al*. Circumferential ultrasound ablation for pulmonary vein isolation: analysis of acute and chronic failures. *J Cardiovasc Electrophysiol* 2002; **13**: 957–61.

37 Nitta T, Lee R, Schuessler RB, Boineau JP, Cox JL. Radial approach: a new concept in surgical treatment for atrial fibrillation I. Concept, anatomic and physiologic bases and development of a procedure. *Ann Thorac Surg* 1999; **67**: 27–35.

38 Nitta T, Ishii Y, Ogasawara H *et al*. Initial experience with the radial incision approach for atrial fibrillation. *Ann Thorac Surg* 1999; **68**: 805–10; discussion 811.

39 Nitta T, Lee R, Watanabe H *et al*. Radial approach: a new concept in surgical treatment for atrial fibrillation. II. Electrophysiologic effects and atrial contribution to ventricular filling. *Ann Thorac Surg* 1999; **67**: 36–50.

40 Thomas SP, Nunn GR, Nicholson IA *et al*. Mechanism, localization and cure of atrial arrhythmias occurring after a new intraoperative endocardial radiofrequency ablation procedure for atrial fibrillation. *J Am Coll Cardiol* 2000; **35**: 442–50.

41 Szalay ZA, Skwara W, Pitschner H-F *et al*. Midterm results after the mini-maze procedure. *Eur J Cardiothorac Surg* 1999; **16**: 306–11.

42 Deneke T, Khargi K, Grewe PH *et al*. Left atrial versus bi-atrial Maze operation using intra-operatively cooled-tip radiofrequency ablation in patients undergoing open-heart surgery: safety and efficacy. *J Am Coll Cardiol* 2002; **39**: 1644–50.

43 Kondo N, Takahashi K, Minakawa M, Daitoku K. Left atrial maze procedure: a useful addition to other corrective operations. *Ann Thorac Surg* 2003; **75**: 1490–4.

44 Vevaina SC, Dastur DK, Manghani DK, Shah NA. Changes in atrial biopsies in chronic rheumatic heart disease. II: Muscle fibre reaction. *Pathol Res Pract* 1985; **179**: 600–9.

45 Melo JQ, Neves J, Adragaõ P *et al*. Surgery for atrial fibrillation using radiofrequency catheter ablation: assessment of results at one year. *Eur J Cardiothorac Surg* 1999; **15**: 851–5.

CHAPTER 11

Surgical Ablation Therapy III: Epicardium-Based Catheter Ablation

Marco A. Zenati

As detailed in previous chapters, intraoperative catheter ablation is under evaluation as a means to replace the cut-and-sew lesion backbone of the classical Maze procedure. Several different energy sources have been reported [1]. As detailed in Chapter 10, the most common site for intraoperative ablation energy application has been the atrial endocardium. Endocardium-based ablation, however, has several limitations, including collateral damage, the need for cardiopulmonary bypass, the potential for endocardial disruption, and inconsistent lesion transmurality. We will review each of these items in detail.

- *Collateral damage.* There is significant potential for unintended injury to contiguous extra-atrial structures, including the esophagus, bronchi, phrenic nerve, pulmonary parenchyma and coronary arteries. Endocardial application of radiofrequency (RF) energy has been associated with esophageal perforation and atrial–enteric fistulae, a grave complication [2, 3]. Coronary artery and phrenic nerve damage have also been reported [4].
- *Need for cardiopulmonary bypass.* Endocardial ablation mandates the use of cardiopulmonary bypass, ischemic cardiac arrest and requires atriotomies in order to reach the target site for ablation. Access can be achieved with a 'minimally invasive' technique: Kottkamp and colleagues used femoral arterial and venous cannulation for cardiopulmonary bypass, a right mini-thoracotomy and aortic cross-clamping through an accessory port to perform a radiofrequency modified Maze [5].
- *Potential for endocardial disruption.* Excessive charring of the endocardium during ablation energy application can lead to thrombus formation, with attendant embolic risk.
- *Inconsistent lesion transmurality.* A critical factor in determining ablation energy requirement is wall thickness, which is quite variable in the human atrium [6, 7]. At present, there is no reliable way to discern atrial wall thickness intraoperatively. Ultrasound may be useful in this regard.

In the last few years, there has been an accelerating development effort in the area of intraoperative epicardium-based ablation [8]. In theory, this approach would permit ablation to be performed in a closed, beating heart

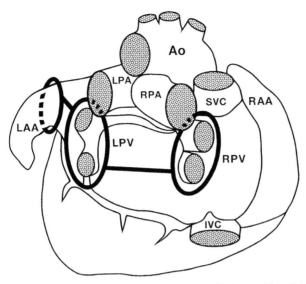

Fig. 11.1 Left atrial lesion set ('mini-maze') for ablation of atrial fibrillation. LAA = left atrial appendage; LPV = left pulmonary veins; RPV = right pulmonary veins; RPA = right pulmonary artery; Ao = aorta; IVC = inferior vena cava; SVC = superior vena cava; RAA = right atrial appendage.

(Fig. 11.1). However, there are significant technical challenges to this approach. Prominent among these are epicardial fat, which in certain regions can be quite prominent, and the fact that blood flowing in the atrial chamber creates a thermal homeostatic effect which makes it very difficult to achieve lethal temperature transmurally during energy application using a single, passively applied ablation electrode. A major technological development has been 'bipolar' ablation devices, with which myocardium targeted for ablation is physically clamped and squeezed between anode and cathode. Devices are currently available from AtriCure (Fig. 11.2; Bipolar RF Clamp, AtriCure, Inc., West Chester, OH, USA) and Medtronic (Fig. 11.3; Cardioblate BP™, Medtronic Inc., Minneapolis, MN, USA).

AtriCure received FDA approval for general surgical use of its device in 2001. In this system, the anodal and cathodal electrodes reside in the jaws of an atraumatic clamp; the jaws are rigid and mounted at a 90° angle with the long axis of the device. The operator depresses a foot pedal and RF energy is delivered to the tissue between the jaws of the clamp at 75 volts and 750 milliamps. The RF generator monitors voltage, current, temperature, time and tissue conductance. Energy delivery is continued until tissue conductance between electrodes in the jaws of the clamp decreases and reaches a steady state, which is maintained for 2 seconds. The design of the clamp is well suited

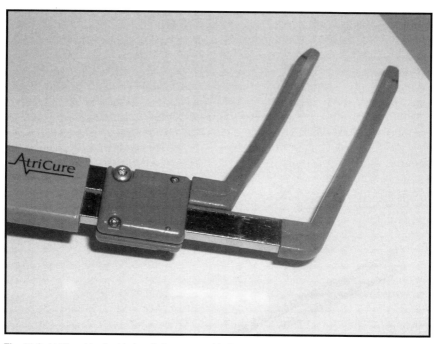

Fig. 11.2 AtriCure bipolar 'dry' radiofrequency ablation device (with permission from AtriCure, West Chester, OH, USA).

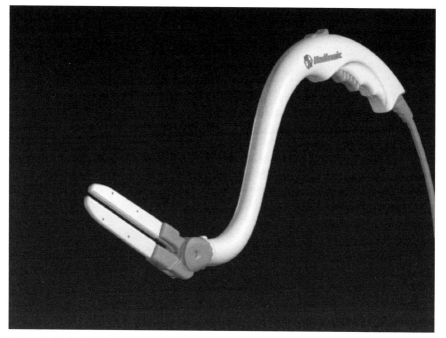

Fig. 11.3 Cardioblate BP (Medtronic, Minneapolis, MN, USA) irrigated bipolar radiofrequency surgical ablation system (with permission from Medtronic).

to encircling the pulmonary veins. For epicardial closed-heart pulmonary vein isolation on the beating heart, the pericardial reflection around the superior and inferior vena cava is dissected, thus allowing mobilization. The right superior pulmonary vein is then dissected from the right main pulmonary artery, paying close attention not to injure or perforate the posterior left atrium, as this maneuver is done in a blind fashion. Once the right superior and inferior pulmonary veins have been dissected, a length of rubber tubing is passed around the veins and the tip of the lower jaw of the clamp is fitted into the opening so that the clamp can easily slide around the posterior veins without risk of further injury to the left atrium; the initial ablation is usually performed with the open jaws of the clamp directed cephalad toward the right pulmonary artery. The rubber tubing is removed and the clamp is adjusted so as to capture within the jaws as much atrium as possible, in order to reduce the chance of creating pulmonary vein stenosis, an occurrence that has been reported in 1–4% of percutaneous RF ablations [9]. Alternatively, the clamp can be placed directly around the pulmonary veins. As the clamp is closed, care is taken to prevent tissue from extruding beyond the tip of the clamp or from folding or bunching up within the jaws. The foot-pedal is depressed and RF energy is delivered. When the generator emits a chirping sound, conductance is low and the ablation is complete within 10–30 seconds. For small pulmonary veins, a single application may be sufficient; however, most patients with permanent atrial fibrillation and enlarged left atrium require a second application, this time starting cephalad and engaging the right superior pulmonary vein first, in order to create an overlapping lesion with the previous. This maneuver creates the potential for a posterior ablation gap, as the intended overlap is not under the direct vision of the surgeon.

We recently performed an evaluation of the AtriCure device in a porcine model [10]. Ablation was performed quickly, with a high rate of success and without complications, and yielded exclusion of a large territory of myocardium. Other investigators have confirmed these data [11, 12]. Gillinov and colleagues recently reported their experience with the AtriCure device in 120 patients [13]. Lesion sets varied as the device was used for pulmonary vein isolation, creation of right atrial lesions or both. There were no device-related complications. Initial incomplete pulmonary vein isolation was uncommon, occurring only with very thick atrium and when tightening of the clamp caused tissue to become folded upon itself or to extrude beyond the jaws of the clamp. In such cases, reapplication of energy produced success.

Medtronic received FDA approval for general surgical use of its device in 2003. The Medtronic device consists of a handheld surgical clamp and an electrical generator. The clamp contains two bipolar electrodes embedded in apposing malleable jaws mounted on an articulated, rotating platform that provides approximately 90° of flexion away from the long axis orientation and 300° of axial rotation (Figs 11.3 and 11.4). Each electrode is fabricated from a stainless steel wire mounted in a porous polymer base that delivers uniform RF energy along its entire length. During energy transfer, the electrode

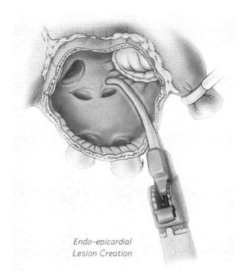

Endo-epicardial
Lesion Creation

Fig. 11.4 Creation of the connecting lesion between the right and left inferior pulmonary veins with the Cardioblate BP (Medtronic, Minneapolis, MN, USA) RF ablation device (with permission from Medtronic).

is continuously irrigated through the porous polymer with normal saline (4–5 ml/min) supplied from an external pressurized source. A proprietary transmurality feedback program within the RF generator monitors tissue impedance between the electrodes and varies the power delivery over the time course of the ablation according to a preset algorithm. Ablation is terminated when the transmurality feedback program detects a steady-state plateau in tissue impedance, indicating full-thickness ablation. As opposed to 'dry' RF, where the greatest amount of heating is concentrated at the tissue surface, potentially causing microbubbles (boiling of intracellular fluid) in the tissue and an associated rise in tissue impedance, irrigated RF ablation cools the surface tissue and lowers the impedance at the tissue–electrode interface, potentially creating a deeper lesion [14]. Hammer and colleagues evaluated the Medtronic device in fresh, excised porcine hearts and noted consistent lesion transmurality [15]. Our group evaluated this device in the same model as that used to evaluate the AtriCure device [16]. As for the AtriCure device, lesions were consistently associated with conduction block, and there was no evidence of atrial endocardial disruption. Thus far, there have been no substantive reports of clinical outcomes associated with its use.

In summary, epicardium-based ablation of AF is undergoing rapid development. The rapidity, simplicity, safety and high rate of lesion success associated with bipolar technology promise to extend the number of patients to whom therapy can be applied. Clinical experience with this technology is nascent and its optimal use in the development of modified Maze procedures remains to be determined.

References

1 Viola N, Williams MR, Oz MC, Ad N. The technology in use for the surgical ablation of atrial fibrillation. *Semin Thorac Cardiovasc Surg* 2002; **14**: 198–205.

2 Gillinov AM, Petterson G, Rice TW. Esophageal injury during radiofrequency ablation of atrial fibrillation. *J Thorac Cardiovasc Surg* 2001; **122**: 1239–40.

3 Doll N, Borger MA, Fabricius A *et al.* Esophageal perforation during left atrial radiofrequency ablation: is the risk too high? *J Thorac Cardiovasc Surg* 2003; **125**: 836–42.

4 Fayad G, Modine T, Le Tourneau T *et al.* Circumflex artery stenosis induced by intraoperative radiofrequency ablation. *Ann Thorac Surg* 2003; **76**: 1291–3.

5 Kottkamp H, Hindricks G, Autschbach R *et al.* Specific linear left atrial lesions in atrial fibrillation: intraoperative radiofrequency ablation using minimally invasive surgical techniques. *J Am Coll Cardiol* 2002; **40**: 475–80.

6 Santiago T, Melo J, Gouvela RH *et al.* Epicardial radiofrequency applications: in vitro and in vivo studies on human atrial myocardium. *Eur J Cardiothorac Surg* 2003; **24**: 481–6.

7 Grubb NR, Furniss S. Science, medicine and the future: radiofrequency ablation for atrial fibrillation. *Br Med J* 2001; **322**: 777–80.

8 Cox JL. Atrial fibrillation II: rationale for surgical treatment. *J Thorac Cardiovasc Surg* 2003; **126**: 1693–9.

9 Robbins IM, Colvin EV, Doyle TP *et al.* Pulmonary vein stenosis after catheter ablation of atrial fibrillation. *Circulation* 1998; **98**: 1769–75.

10 Schwartzman D, Bonanomi G, Zenati MA. Epicardium-based left atrial ablation: impact on electromechanical properties. *J Cardiovasc Electrophysiol* 2003; **14**: 1–6.

11 Prasad SM, Maniar HS, Moustakidis P *et al.* Epicardial ablation on the beating heart: progress towards an off-pump Maze procedure. *Heart Surg Forum* 2001; **5**: 100–4.

12 Prasad SM, Maniar HS, Schuessler RB, Damiano RJ. Chronic transmural atrial ablation by using bipolar radiofrequency energy on the beating heart. *J Thorac Cardiovasc Surg* 2002; **124**: 708–13.

13 Gillinov AM, McCarthy PM. Atricure bipolar radiofrequency clamp for intraoperative ablation of atrial fibrillation. *Ann Thorac Surg* 2002; **74**: 2165–8.

14 Demazumder D, Mirotznik MS, Schwartzman D. Biophysics of radiofrequency ablation using an irrigated electrode. *J Intervent Cardiac Electrophysiol* 2001; **5**: 377–89.

15 Hammer CE, Lutterman A, Potter DD *et al.* Irrigated bipolar radiofrequency ablation with transmurality feedback for the surgical Cox-Maze procedure. *Heart Surg Forum* 2003; **6**: 418–23.

16 Bonanomi G, Schwartzman D, Francischelli D, Hebsgaard K, Zenati MA. A new device for beating heart bipolar radiofrequency atrial ablation. *J Thorac Cardiovasc Surg* 2003; **126**: 1859–66.

CHAPTER 12

Modification of the Left Atrial Appendage

Marco A. Zenati, David Schwartzman

Cardioembolism is the major cause of disability and death which can be clearly attributed to atrial fibrillation (AF), particularly in the elderly [1–6]. Systemic anticoagulation with warfarin has been demonstrated as an effective means of reducing the rate of AF-attributable cardioembolism [2, 7, 8]. However, proper compliance with this drug is difficult, and complications associated with even proper use are common, particularly in the elderly [6, 9]. In addition, its use is commonly contraindicated [10]. The aggregate effect is that warfarin is used in fewer than 50% of AF patients for whom a favorable risk–benefit ratio exists [3, 10]. Although effective, warfarin is imperfect in preventing AF-attributable cardioembolism [8].

Autopsy and echocardiographic studies in AF patients have clearly shown that left atrial thrombus, when present, is vastly more common in the left atrial appendage (LAA) than elsewhere, and that the LAA plays the central role in AF-attributable cardioembolism (Table 12.1) [11–19]. The LAA has several properties that could explain this [20]. First, it is a *cul de sac*, which results in flow stasis relative to other regions of the LA. Secondly, it is trabeculated and lobulated, which creates a number of dead-end, narrow passages, a further substrate for stasis. Finally, the tissue comprising the LAA is unique and may form a biochemical substrate more favorable to coagulation factor activation.

The anatomy of the LAA lends itself to surgical modification, which we define as occlusion of the orifice with or without resection of distal myocardium. It is an elongated pouch with a narrow entry (orifice) and its location on the free wall of the left atrium renders it accessible to surgical access, with or without thoracotomy. This gives practical momentum to the hypothesis that elimination of the LAA substrate would be a non-pharmacological means of removing AF-attributable cardioembolic risk [19, 20]. The LAA has been the target for modification during open-chest, non-arrhythmia surgery for years, and there are passionate advocates for its routine use in this setting, independent of AF history [21, 22]. As detailed in previous chapters, it is standard during the Maze procedure. Whether by stapling or oversewing, modification of the appendage can be performed quickly and does not add to procedural morbidity. Quality control is critical, as recent reports have demonstrated postoperative orifice patency; this will be discussed in more

Table 12.1 Review of published reports detailing the frequency and site of left atrial thrombus location in patients with non-rheumatic AF (modified from Blackshear *et al.* [19])

Setting	Number of patients	Thrombus location		Reference
		LA appendage	LA cavity	
TEE*	317	66	1	18
TEE	233	34	1	14
Autopsy	506	35	12	11
TEE	52	2	2	12
TEE	48	12	1	13
TEE and operation	171	8	3	14
ACUTE	549	67	9**	15
TEE	272	19	0	16
TEE	60	6	0	17
Total	1288	249	29	

LA = left atrium; ACUTE = Assessment of Cardioversion Using Transesophageal Echocardiography Multicenter Trial; TEE = transesophageal echocardiography.
*Five percent of patients in this trial had mitral stenosis or prosthetic mitral valve.
**Calculated by deduction of left atrial appendage thrombi from all left heart thrombi.

detail below. This observation, combined with the absence of efficacy data and recent treatises which emphasize the potential importance of the LAA in mechanical, biochemical and neurological function, have tempered enthusiasm for its routine use [20, 23–30]. As a matter of fact, there are as yet no reports of an appropriately controlled study detailing the structural and functional repercussions of LAA modification in man.

Classical techniques for open-chest LAA modification are neck ligation, purse string occlusion, and stapling [31–33]. Ligation and purse string are the most widely used techniques and are associated with a low incidence of complications. Stapling is a reasonable alternative, especially for patients with a wide LAA orifice [32]. The main risk of these methods is atrial tear, the incidence of which is under 1% in experienced hands, and which can be readily treated intraoperatively [21]. We are not aware of any reports of postoperative mischief related to tearing at an LAA modification site.

As mentioned above, recent reports have emphasized the need for quality control of these techniques. In a prospective evaluation using early postoperative transesophageal echocardiography, Katz and colleagues demonstrated that in 36% of patients undergoing concomitant mitral valve surgery, LAA modification was incomplete [34]. In terms of cardioembolic risk, the 'partially occluded' LAA substrate may be even worse than the native state. Long-term imaging studies in patients after LAA modification are completely lacking. Given these data, it seems reasonable in the least to image patients early after LAA modification to ensure complete anatomical success. If lacking, it may be reasonable to reinstitute warfarin therapy, at least until subsequent study was to demonstrate progression to complete occlusion.

If LAA modification is indeed an effective non-pharmacological technique for prevention of AF-attributable cardioembolism, its application would overwhelmingly be in patients who had no need for concomitant cardiac surgery. This fact has driven the development of new, less invasive methods for LAA modification. Several years ago, successful LAA modification in humans was demonstrated without thoracotomy, via thoracoscopic access [31, 35]. However, breach of the pleural space and the requirement for general anesthesia would limit widespread application of this technique. We recently demonstrated the feasibility of LAA modification using an epicardial approach performed via percutaneous subxiphoid access, which does not breach the pleural space and which therefore might be performed without general anesthesia, on an ambulatory basis [36]. Other investigators have conceptualized a percutaneous, catheter-based endocardial approach in which a prosthetic device is delivered to occupy and effectively occlude the LAA [37]. Interim data in small numbers of patients demonstrate the feasibility of this technique [38]. In summary, LAA modification is feasible, but safety and efficacy issues remain to be elucidated. If these issues are resolved favorably, this could have a major impact on AF patient management. It can be reasonably stated that, if the cardioembolic risk attributable to AF were to be removed, the disease for the vast majority of patients would be reduced to a mere annoyance.

References

1 Benjamin EJ, Levy D, Vaziri EM *et al*. Independent risk factors for atrial fibrillation in a population-based cohort: the Framingham Heart Study. *JAMA* 1994; **271**: 840–4.

2 Goldstein LB, Adams R, Becker K *et al*. Primary prevention of ischemic stroke: A statement for healthcare professionals from the Stroke Council of the American Heart Association. *Stroke* 2001; **32**: 280–99.

3 Lamassa M, Di Carlo A, Pracucci G *et al*. Characteristics, outcome, and care of stroke associated with atrial fibrillation in Europe: data from a multicenter multinational, hospital-based registry. *Stroke* 2001; **32**: 392–8.

4 Albers GW, Dalen JE, Laupacis A *et al*. Antithrombotic therapy in atrial fibrillation. *Chest* 2001; **119**: 194S–206S.

5 Wolf PA, Abbot RD, Kannel WB. Atrial fibrillation as an independent risk factor for stroke: the Framingham Study. *Stroke* 1991; **22**: 983–8.

6 Wolf PA, Abbot RD, Kannel WB. Atrial fibrillation: a major contributor to stroke in the elderly. *Arch Intern Med* 1987; **147**: 1561–4.

7 Fuster V, Ryden LE, Asinger RW *et al*. ACC/AHA/ESC Guidelines for the Management of Patients with Atrial Fibrillation: Executive Summary. *J Am Coll Cardiol* 2001; **38**: 2118–50.

8 Hart RG. Antithrombotic therapy to prevent stroke in patients with atrial fibrillation: a meta-analysis. *Ann Intern Med* 1999; **131**: 492–501.

9 Laupacis A. Antithrombotic therapy in atrial fibrillation. *Chest* 1998; **114**: 579S–589S.

10 Bungard TJ, Ghali WA, Teo KK, McAlister FA, Tsuyuki RT. Why do patients with atrial fibrillation not receive warfarin? *Arch Intern Med* 2000; **160**: 41–6.

11 Alberg H. Atrial fibrillation 1: a study of atrial thrombosis and systemic embolism in a necropsy material. *Acta Medica Scandinavica* 1969; **1185**: 373–9.

12 Tsai LM, Chen JH, Lin LJ, Yang YJ. Role of transesophageal echocardiography in detecting left atrial thrombus and spontaneous echo contrast in patients with mitral valve disease or non-rheumatic atrial fibrillation. *J Formos Med Assoc* 1990; **89**: 270–4.

13 Brown J, Sadler DB. Left atrial thrombi in non-rheumatic atrial fibrillation: assessment of prevalence by transesophageal echocardiography. *Int J Card Imaging* 1993; **9**: 65–72.

14 Manning W, *et al*. Sensitivity and specificity of transesophageal echo for left atrial thrombi: a prospective, consecutive surgical study. *Circulation* 1994; **90**: 1202a.

15 Klein AL, Grimm RA, Murray RD *et al*. Use of transesophageal echocardiography to guide cardioversion in patients with atrial fibrillation. *N Engl J Med* 2001; **344**: 1411–20.

16 Leung DY, Black IW, Cranney GB, Hopkins AP, Walsh WF. Prognostic implications of left atrial spontaneous echo contrast in nonvalvular atrial fibrillation. *J Am Coll Cardiol* 1994; **24**: 755–62.

17 Hart RG, Halperin JL. Atrial fibrillation and stroke. Revisiting the dilemmas. *Stroke* 1994; **25**: 1337–41.

18 Stoddard MF, Dawkins PR, Prince CR, Ammash NM. Left atrial appendage thrombus is not uncommon in patients with acute atrial fibrillation and a recent embolic event: a transesophageal echocardiographic study. *J Am Coll Cardiol* 1995; **25**: 452–9.

19 Blackshear JL, Odell JA. Appendage obliteration to reduce stroke in cardiac surgical patients with atrial fibrillation. *Ann Thorac Surg* 1996; **61**: 755–9.

20 Al-Saady NM, Obel OA, Camm AJ. Left atrial appendage: structure, function and role in thromboembolism. *Heart* 1999; **82**: 547–54.

21 Johnson WD. The left atrial appendage: our most lethal human attachment! *Eur J Cardiothorac Surg* 2000; **17**: 718–22.

22 Frye RL, Kronmal R, Schaff HV, Myers WO, Gersh BJ. Stroke in coronary artery bypass graft surgery: an analysis of the CASS experience. The participants in the Coronary Artery Surgery Study. *Int J Cardiol* 1992; **36**: 213–21.

23 Stewart JM, Dean R, Brown M *et al*. Bilateral atrial appendectomy abolishes increased plasma atrial natriuretic peptide release and blunts sodium and water excretion during volume loading in conscious dogs. *Circ Res* 1992; **70**: 724–32.

24 Cox JL. Successful surgical treatment of atrial fibrillation. Review and clinical update. *JAMA* 1991; **266**: 1976–80.

25 Yoshihara F, Nishikimi T, Sasako Y *et al*. Preservation of right atrial appendage improves reduced plasma atrial natriuretic peptide levels after the maze procedure. *J Thorac Cardiovasc Surg* 2000; **119**: 790–4.

26 Amano J, Suzuki A, Sunamori M *et al*. Alteration of atrial natriuretic peptide response to sodium loading after cardiac operation. *J Thorac Cardiovasc Surg* 1995; **110**: 75–80.

27 Omari BO, Nelson RJ, Robertson JM. Effect of right atrial appendectomy on the release of atrial natriuretic hormone. *J Thorac Cardiovasc Surg* 1991; **102**: 272–9.

28 Zimmerman MB, Blaine EH, Stricker EM. Water intake in hypovolemic sheep: effects of crushing the left atrial appendage. *Science* 1981; **211**: 489–91.

29 Massoudy P, Beblo S, Raschke P, Zahler S, Becker BF *et al*. Influence of intact left atrial appendage on hemodynamic parameters of isolated guinea pig heart. *Eur J Med Res* 1998; **3**: 470–4.

30 Hoit BD, Shao Y, Tsai LM *et al*. Altered left atrial compliance after atrial appendectomy. Influence on left atrial and ventricular filling. *Circ Res* 1993; **72**: 167–75.

31 Johnson WD. Method for closing an atrial appendage. Patent 5306234, 1993.

32 Landymore R, Kinley CE. Staple closure of the left atrial appendage. *Can J Surg* 1984; **27**: 144–5.

33 DiSesa VJ, Tam S, Cohn LH. Ligation of the left atrial appendage using an automatic surgical stapler. *Ann Thorac Surg* 1988; **46**: 652–3.

34 Katz ES, Tsiamtsiouris T, Applebaum RM. Surgical left atrial appendage ligation is frequently incomplete: a transesophageal echocardiographic study. *J Am Coll Cardiol* 2000; **36**: 468–71.

35 Odell JA, Blackshear JL, Davies E *et al.* Thoracoscopic obliteration of the left atrial appendage: potential for stroke reduction? *Ann Thorac Surg* 1996; **61**: 565–9.

36 Zenati M, Schwartzman D, Gartner M, McKeel D. Feasibility of a new method for percutaneous occlusion of the left atrial appendage. *Circulation* 2002; **106**: II-619.

37 Sievert H, Lesh MD, Trepels T *et al.* Percutaneous left atrial appendage transcatheter occlusion to prevent stroke in high-risk patients with atrial fibrillation – early clinical experience. *Circulation* 2002; **105**: 1887–9.

38 Hannah IR, Kolm P, Martin R *et al.* Left atrial structure and function after percutaneous left atrial appendage transcatheter occlusion (PLAATO). *J Am Coll Cardiol* 2004; **43**: 1868–72.

PART III

Potential Areas of Opportunity for AF Management

CHAPTER 13

Transpericardial Therapy

Michael R. Ujhelyi

Long-term systemic pharmacotherapy for rhythm control of atrial fibrillation (AF) is generally not feasible, because of limitations of inefficacy, intolerance and safety, each of which is associated with exposure of non-atrial tissue to the drug. A means to preferentially deliver a drug to atrial tissue may thus improve its clinical utility. The utility of intrathecal pharmacotherapy is evidence of the feasibility of chronic regional drug delivery. Like the brain, the heart is surrounded by a biologically active reservoir, the pericardium. In this chapter we explore the possibility of using the pericardial space as a vehicle for chronic atrial pharmacotherapy in man.

Pericardial anatomy and physiology

The pericardium is comprised of an outer fibrous envelope and an inner serous layer. The serous pericardium is composed of two layers, parietal and visceral [1]. The pericardial fluid space (PFS) is located between these layers. The parietal layer is attached to the fibrous pericardium and is hence separated from the myocardium. The visceral layer is in direct contact with the epicardium. The pericardial fluid space is continuous, except at the pericardial reflections (great vessels and pulmonary vein regions). A network of sinuses permits direct access of pericardial fluid to myocardial regions even in the reflection zones. The volume of the PFS is generally believed to be 20–25 ml (0.25 ± 15 ml/kg) [1]. Dye studies suggest that pericardial fluid is not uniformly distributed within the PFS. Specifically, most of the fluid volume resides within the atrial-ventricular and inter-ventricular grooves and the sinuses. Pharmacokinetic studies suggest that there is continuous mixing of fluid throughout the PFS, so that fluid content is spatially uniform [2–4]. Typically, the pericardial fluid is composed of extracellular fluid and is in constant diffusion equilibrium with epicardial tissue [5, 6]. However, pericardial or cardiac diseases can significantly alter fluid content [7]. For example, patients with active ischemia have much higher levels of basic fibroblast growth factor and vascular endothelial growth factor, which may be associated with angiogenesis and neovascularization [8, 9]. Similarly, left ventricular failure can be associated with marked elevation in pericardial fluid endothelin levels that are up to 200-fold greater than plasma endothelin levels, which is associated with reduction in global coronary blood flow and the development of ventricular arrhythmias [10].

Accessing the pericardial fluid space

In addition to thoracotomy, several techniques have been used to access the PFS, including thoracoscopy, subxiphoid puncture and transmyocardial puncture. The latter two techniques are of particular interest regarding stand-alone intrapericardial pharmacotherapy: they do not breach the pleural space and can be done without incision, and thus could be performed on an ambulatory basis. In the subxiphoid approach, entry to the PFS occurs near the apex of the right ventricle. Recently, tools have been developed to enhance efficiency and reduce the risk associated with the traditional open-needle technique [11, 12]. Subxiphoid access is used clinically for procedures such as myocardial ablation and injection. In the transmyocardial approach, entry into the PFS is achieved via needle puncture of the right atrial appendage [13]. This approach has the theoretical advantage of not breaching the fibrous pericardial wall, which could result in leakage. There are no reports of its use in humans. Regardless of access method, the development of a technique for intrapericardial pharmacotherapy will require chronic pericardial access and the presence of a foreign body, such as a drug delivery catheter. Concerns regarding this include inflammation, infection and catheter malfunction [14]. To date, we are unaware of clinical or animal data demonstrating long-term tolerability of a relatively large mass of foreign material, such as a catheter, in the pericardial space.

Pericardial fluid pharmacokinetics

Removal of compounds from pericardial fluid occurs via lymphatics and the epicardial vasculature [15]. Certain compounds may be enzymatically transformed prior to removal. The kinetics of a given compound probably depends upon multiple factors, including molecular size, tissue affinity, water solubility and enzymatic stability. Large molecules such as proteins are slowly cleared from the pericardial space, perhaps via lymphatics, yielding a duration of activity which exceeds that in plasma after intravenous administration [4, 16]. For example, the duration of activity of atrial natriuretic peptide in pericardial fluid after direct administration markedly exceeds that in plasma after intravenous administration [16]. A similar phenomenon has been observed with 5-fluorouracil (Fig. 13.1) [3]. An additional observation, which is a key conceptual element toward transpericardial AF pharmacotherapy, was the ultralow plasma level of drug throughout the course of intrapericardial therapy [3]. In contrast, small, water-soluble compounds introduced directly into pericardial fluid may have an abbreviated duration of activity relative to plasma after intravenous administration. For example, procainamide has a pericardial fluid half-life ranging from 30 to 41 minutes, compared with a

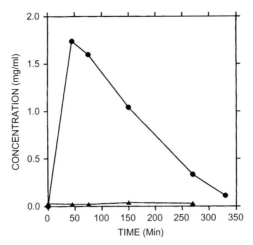

Fig. 13.1 Concentration–time curve of 5-fluorouracil for pericardial fluid (circles) and plasma (triangles) after a pericardial injection of 200 mg 5-fluorouracil. (Reprinted from *Cancer Chemotherapy and Pharmacology*, 40, Lerner-Tung *et al.*, Pharmacokinetics of intrapericardial adminstration of 5-flourouracil, 318–20, Copyright 1997, with permission from Springer-verlag [3].)

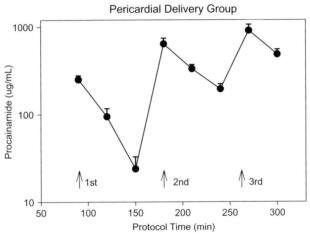

Fig. 13.2 Line graph depicting pericardial (closed circles) procainamide concentrations for pericardial procainamide doses of 0.5, 1 and 2 mg/kg (first, second and third doses respectively). There were no detectable plasma concentrations. (Reprinted and adapted from *Journal of Cardiovascular Electrophysiology*, 13, Vjhelyi *et al.*, Intrapericardial therapeutics: a pharmacodynamic and pharmacokinetic comparison between pericardial and intravenous procainamide, 605–11, Copyright 2002, with permission from Blackwell Publishing Ltd [2].)

180-minute plasma half-life (Fig. 13.2) [17]. As noted above, despite its rapid removal from pericardial fluid and longer half-life in plasma, peak plasma levels were always unmeasurable because of the low loading dose required to achieve therapeutic pericardial fluid levels [17]. As might be expected, movement of molecules across the pericardial barrier is not unidirectional.

For example, intravenously administered procainamide rapidly diffuses into the pericardial space across a plasma-to-pericardial fluid concentration gradient such that pericardial fluid concentrations rapidly reach equilibrium (Figs 13.3 and 13.4).

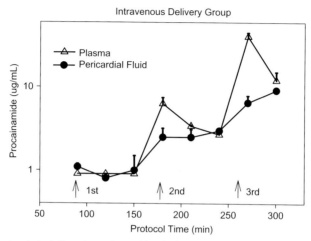

Fig. 13.3 Line graph depicting plasma (open triangles) and pericardial (closed circles) concentrations of procainamide after intravenous procainamide delivery doses of 2, 8 and 16 mg/kg (first, second and third doses respectively). (Reprinted and adapted from *Journal of Cardiovascular Electrophysiology*, 13, Vjhelyi *et al.*, Intrapericardial therapeutics: a pharmacodynamic and pharmacokinetic comparison between pericardial and intravenous procainamide, 605–11, Copyright 2002, with permission from Blackwell Publishing Ltd [2].)

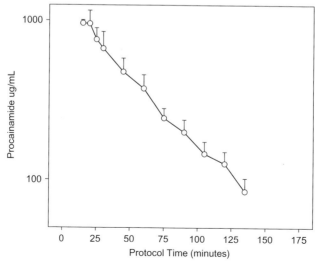

Fig. 13.4 Line graph of pericardial fluid procainamide concentration–time profile after a single 2 mg/kg procainamide pericardial dose study.

Regional considerations

Although there are no detailed reports, it is clear that delivery of molecules from pericardial fluid to tissues contiguous to the pericardium is regionally non-uniform. The combined effects of mass, thickness and a dense overlying vasculature serve to shield the ventricular myocardium relative to the atrial myocardium as well as the epicardial coronary artery and neural tissues [2]. Disproportionate myocardial delivery favoring the atrium is another important conceptual element toward the transpericardial pharmacotherapy of AF. Moreno and colleagues demonstrated this phenomenon in a study in which esmolol, directly instilled into the PFS, had an 'atrium preferred' effect (profound reduction in sinus rate without change in ventricular inotropy). This was in contrast to the effect after intravenous administration [18]. Of course, it may be difficult to distinguish atrial effect from direct effects on contiguous neural tissue and/or the neural–myocardial interface. Ayers and colleagues measured regional myocardial amiodarone concentrations after intrapericardial administration [19]. Atrium and ventricular epicardium had the highest concentrations; ventricular endocardial concentrations were approximately 10-fold lower. It is important to note that regional differences in myocardial concentration may or may not translate into a regionally disparate effect. For example, high pericardial concentrations of procainamide produce no effect on left ventricular endocardial refractory periods, whereas amiodarone produces more symmetrical prolongations endocardially and epicardially [2, 19]. As detailed above, specific properties of individual drugs will dictate this behavior.

Developmental experience

Several studies have addressed the impact of transpericardial pharmacotherapy on atrial electrophysiological properties. Labhasetwar and colleagues demonstrated that ibutilide delivered as an intrapericardial pacing lead-based polymer can alter atrial refractoriness transmurally and diminish the likelihood of AF induction [20]. Ayers and colleagues, using intrapericardial amiodarone injected into the PFS, demonstrated similar results [19]. We performed a sequential (escalating), acute, single-bolus study comparing intravenous and intrapericardially administered procainamide. We observed that a 2 mg/kg dose injected into the PFS increased the right atrial refractory period in excess of 20%; this effect was sustained for at least 90 minutes after a pericardial dose. In contrast, a 2-mg/kg intravenous procainamide dose had no effect on refractory period; a dose of between 10 and 18 mg/kg was needed to achieve an effect equivalent to transpericardial administration. A follow-up study provided better insight into the pharmacodynamic response of a single 2-mg/kg procainamide dose delivered transpericardially. Pericardial procainamide significantly increased atrial refractory period by 20% (180 ± 8 to 216 ± 16 ms, $P < 0.001$), similar to the sequential dose study (Fig. 13.5). Maximum

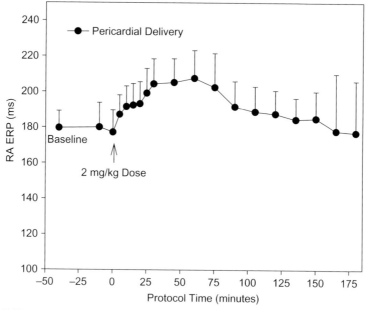

Fig. 13.5 Line graph depicting right atrial effective refractory period versus protocol time.

prolongation of refractory period occurred 48 ± 6 minutes after administration; the effect completely resolved at 90–120 minutes (Fig. 13.6). Importantly, no changes in ventricular electrophysiological parameters were noted at any interval. In addition, in contrast to intravenous administration, transpericardial therapy was not associated with hemodynamic intolerance (diminishment in left ventricular contractility, vasodilatation).

Another promising route in the development of transpericardial pharmacosuppression of AF may include the targeting of contiguous neural structures. As is discussed in detail in Chapter 2, it is clear that AF triggering is a neurologically mediated event. Several investigators have demonstrated that manipulation of cardiac sympathovagal balance can be achieved using transpericardial pharmacotherapy. In a rabbit model, Dorward and colleagues demonstrated that pericardial installation of a local neural conduction blocking agent (procaine) produced complete blockade of cardiac vagal and sympathetic efferent activity, as assessed by reflex responses to nitroglycerin and phenylephrine [21]. These effects were significantly greater in magnitude and duration relative to those observed after intravenous dosing of the same drug. Additional data demonstrated that pericardial installation of hexamethonium and tetrodotoxin each produced vagolysis, while only tetrodotoxin produced sympatholysis [21]. In a pig model, Gleason and colleagues compared AF inducibility after transpericardial or intravenous procaine therapy [22]. Whereas transpericardial therapy significantly reduced inducibility, no effect

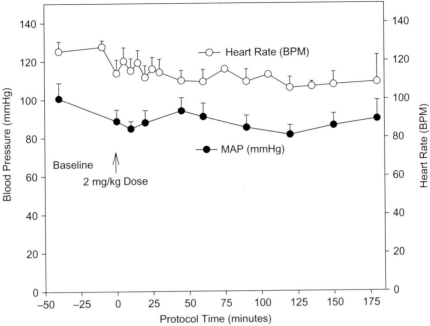

Fig. 13.6 (Left axis) Line graph of aortic blood pressure (mmHg) and heart rate versus protocol time (*P* < 0.0001 versus baseline). (Right axis) Heart rate (beats/minute). MAP = mean arterial pressure. BPM = beats/minute. (Reprinted and adapted from *Journal of Cardiovascular Electrophysiology*, 13, Vjhelyi *et al.*, Intrapericardial therapeutics: a pharmacodynamic and pharmacokinetic comparison between pericardial and intravenous procainamide, 605–11, Copyright 2002, with permission from Blackwell Publishing Ltd [2].)

was noted after intravenous administration. Although not demonstrated in this study, it is conceivable that procaine accumulation in the PFS after intravenous administration is insufficient in quantity and/or access to influence local neural traffic. Important among considerations in the development of transpericardial pharmacosuppression of AF is the electrophysiological impact of this therapy on ventricular tissue. As detailed above, the anatomy and physiology of the ventricle as regards transpericardial therapy make it more likely than the atrium to be heterogeneously exposed. In theory, the resulting electrical heterogeneity can be proarrhythmic. For example, regional ventricular administration of sodium channel blocking drugs can promote the inducibility of ventricular fibrillation in certain animal models [23, 24]. However, in our study using procainamide, transpericardial administration did not promote the inducibility of ventricular fibrillation. We performed a separate study examining transpericardial therapy with ibutilide [25]. Unlike the procainamide study, in this study a canine model of AV block was used. The ventricular arrhythmia susceptibility in this model, unlike healthy animals, is well documented. We demonstrated that, relative to intravenous administration, transpericardial administration of ibutilide was not proarrhythmic (Fig. 13.7).

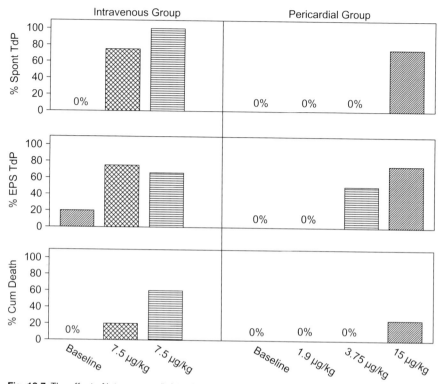

Fig. 13.7 The effect of intravenous (left half) and pericardial (right half) ibutilide delivery on the induction of spontaneous (top panel) and electrically induced (middle panel) arrhythmias and the cumulative death rate (bottom panel) according to dose level.

Chronic transpericardial therapy

So far, transpericardial pharmacotherapy has been practiced using a single dose delivered via a temporary vehicle (catheter). In conceptualizing a clinical role for transpericardial pharmacosuppression of AF, it is possible that continuous or recurrent bolus administration of an agent will be necessary. Indwelling infusion catheters have long been in clinical use for recurrent bolus intravenous pharmacotherapy, such as in oncology applications. However, chronic use is limited by issues of infection and catheter patency. A more attractive concept is the fully implantable drug pump system, with which a drug can be delivered continuously or intermittently (timed or on demand). The system has a reservoir which requires only intermittent refilling (needle puncture of a self-sealing septum), which can be performed in the ambulatory setting. The drug pump system has been used clinically. It is typically placed subcutaneously in the abdomen, with the infusion catheter tunneled to the target organ. There are two main designs of implantable drug delivery devices. The first design uses a fluorocarbon propellant and accurately delivers a drug at a constant flow rate. The advantage of this system is its simplicity, as it lacks electrical components. Each refill recharges the propellant. However, drug dosage changes require a change in drug concentration or catheter size; hence, there is limited flexibility. The second design is a multiprogrammable electrically driven pump. Clinical application of chronic drug pump therapy has included intraspinal (epidural or intrathecal) delivery to manage either chronic refractory spasticity or pain as well as selective intra-arterial therapy for the chemotherapy of primary or metastatic hepatic malignancies. Another use, but an uncommon one, is chronic intravascular (hepatic artery) infusion of floxuridine or methotrexate for the treatment of primary metastatic cancer. Use of the drug pump for chronic transpericardial pharmacotherapy is under evaluation in animal models.

Keys to further development

Although it is a promising concept, transpericardial pharmacotherapy for AF suppression is nascent. From our vantage point, there are several keys for further development.

Improved insight into physiology of the pericardial fluid and the fluid–myocardial interface

Fundamental issues are as yet unexplored. For example, as described above, although the atrium is anatomically well suited to transpericardial therapy, there are only trivial data examining the magnitude and extent of the delivery to atrial tissue of any drug. In addition, as cited above, concepts of pericardial fluid pharmacokinetics are largely derived from models of healthy hearts. It is not clear whether and how structural and functional disease could alter these concepts. For example, it is possible that prior pericardiotomy will produce regional disparities which affect drug delivery. Similarly, it is possible that changes in intraventricular pressure or output will influence pericardial fluid pharmacokinetics or regional delivery patterns.

Clarity as to which pharmacological agents are of interest

As detailed above, the focus thus far has been on drugs with traditional 'anti-arrhythmic' electrophysiological properties. However, different drug classes may be of greater interest. One potentially interesting class involves drugs which influence mechanisms of cardiac self-protection, an example of which is the nitric oxide (NO) system. NO is a central player in ischemic, inflammatory and coagulation pathways, in general exerting a protective influence [26, 27, 28]. Atrial NO levels could conceivably be increased via transpericardial administration. For example, Fei and colleagues demonstrated that L-arginine (an NO precursor) introduced into the PFS made animals more resistant to ischemically mediated ventricular tachyarrhythmias [29]. Nitroglycerin administration produced similar results. Similarly, Baek and colleagues showed that a nitric oxide donor molecule, diazeniumdiolate, administered intrapericardially was successful in preventing stenosis in contiguous (epicardial) coronary arteries after stent implantation [30]. Other drugs which appear to have efficacy in enhancing cardiac self-protection include angiotensin-converting enzyme inhibitors and receptor blockers. Enteral use of these agents has been associated with increasing the resistance of the atrial substrate to AF [31]. It is possible that transpericardial administration will expand the utility of such agents; for example, by permitting large atrial concentrations which could not be achieved and/or would not be tolerated via enteral administration. A second 'class' of drugs of potential interest have activity in myocardial or vascular remodeling. For example, transpericardially administered paclitaxel greatly reduced restenosis in epicardial coronary arteries after injury by inhibiting neointimal proliferation [32]. Matrix metalloproteinase inhibitors are another group of compounds in this class which have the potential to ameliorate the development of atrial structural pathology [33]. A third 'class' of agents with potential promise for transpericardial delivery to the atrium are viral vectors, the contents of which may establish a long-term therapeutic presence. For example, Lazarous and colleagues introduced growth factor gene vectors into PFS and subsequently demonstrated significant and sustained vascular endothelial growth factor gene expression and production [34]. It is possible that direct intrapericardial administration may overcome some of the limitations of tissue-specific transfection encountered during systemic vector administration.

An additional consideration in the development of specific drugs of interest is the potential for their chemical modification to enhance transpericardial use. For example, previous studies have demonstrated that modification of molecular structure can significantly affect activity time after introduction into pericardial fluid. In the study by Baek and colleagues noted above, the NO donor molecule, diazeniumdiolate, was derivatized with bovine serum albumin. This resulted in a five fold increase in pericardial fluid activity time compared with a small NO donor molecule, such as diethylenetriamine [30]. This was a key element in the success of this therapy in preventing stenosis in coronary arteries after stent implantation. Conceptually similar to chemical modifications designed to improve the utility of transpericardial atrial therapy, it is possible that biological alteration will be performed to enhance the targeting of atrial tissue relative to other exposed tissues. For example, viral vectors for gene delivery may be constructed in such a way as to favor atrial infection.

Evidence in support of feasibility of long-term transpericardial therapy

As noted above, clarity as to which agents are to be used in a transpericardial approach is lacking. It is possible that the desired agent will need to be delivered recurrently or continuously. Thus far there is no experience with chronic transpericardial therapy. It is conceivable that access catheters may not be durable, or may engender an inflammatory response which may produce intolerable symptoms or limit drug delivery. As with intravenous therapy, chronic use may not be feasible because of infection. For a given agent, evidence in support of efficacy and safety of long-term transpericardial administration will be necessary.

References

1 Choe YH, Im JG, Park JH, Han MC, Kim CW. The anatomy of the pericardial space: a study in cadavers and patients. *AJR Am J Roentgenol* 1987; **149**: 693–7.

2 Ujhelyi M, Hadsell K, Euler D, Mehra R. Intrapericardial therapeutics: a pharmacodynamic and pharmacokinetic comparison between pericardial and intravenous procainamide. *J Cardiovasc Electrophysiol* 2002; **13**: 605–11.

3 Lerner-Tung MB, Chang AY, Ong LS, Kreiser D. Pharmacokinetics of intrapericardial administration of 5-fluorouracil. *Cancer Chemother Pharmacol* 1997; **40**: 318–20.

4 Stoll HP, Carlson K, Keefer LK, Hrabie JA, March KL. Pharmacokinetics and consistency of pericardial delivery directed to coronary arteries: direct comparison with endoluminal delivery. *Clin Cardiol* 1999; **22**: I10–16.

5 Meyers DG, Bouska DJ. Diagnostic usefulness of pericardial fluid cytology. *Chest* 1989; **95**: 1142–3.

6 Dickson TJ, Gurudutt V, Nguyen AQ *et al.* Establishment of a clinically correlated human pericardial fluid bank: evaluation of intrapericardial diagnostic potential. *Clin Cardiol* 1999; **22**: I40–2.

7 Meyers DG, Meyers RE, Prendergast TW. The usefulness of diagnostic tests on pericardial fluid. *Chest* 1997; **111**: 1213–21.

8 Iwakura A, Fujita M, Hasegawa K *et al.* Pericardial fluid from patients with unstable angina induces vascular endothelial cell apoptosis. *J Am Coll Cardiol* 2000; **35**: 1785–90.

9 Laham RJ, Hung D, Simons M. Therapeutic myocardial angiogenesis using percutaneous intrapericardial drug delivery. *Clin Cardiol* 1999; **22**: I6–9.

10 Horkay F, Szokodi I, Merkely B *et al.* Potential pathophysiologic role of endothelin-1 in canine pericardial fluid. *J Cardiovasc Pharmacol* 1998; **31**: S401–2.

11 Laham RJ, Simons M, Hung D. Subxyphoid access of the normal pericardium: a novel drug delivery technique. *Catheter Cardiovasc Interv* 1999; **47**: 109–11.

12 Seferovic PM, Ristic AD, Maksimovic R *et al.* Initial clinical experience with PerDUCER device: promising new tool in the diagnosis and treatment of pericardial disease. *Clin Cardiol* 1999; **22**: I30–5.

13 Waxman S, Pulerwitz TC, Rowe KA, Quist WC, Verrier RL. Preclinical safety testing of percutaneous transatrial access to the normal pericardial space for local cardiac drug delivery and diagnostic sampling. *Catheter Cardiovasc Interv* 2000; **49**: 472–7.

14 Fioravanti J, Buzzard CJ, Harris JP. Pericardial effusion and tamponade as a result of percutaneous silastic catheter use. *Neonatal Netw* 1998; **17**: 39–42.

15 Hollenberg M, Dougherty J. Lymph flow and 131-I-albumin resorption from pericardial effusions in man. *Am J Cardiol* 1969; **24**: 514–22.

16 Szokodi I, Horkay F, Kiss P *et al.* Characterization and stimuli for production of pericardial fluid atrial natriuretic peptide in dogs. *Life Sci* 1997; **61**: 1349–59.

17 Nolan PE. Pharmacokinetics and pharmacodynamics of intravenous agents for ventricular arrhythmias. *Pharmacotherapy* 1997; **17**: 65S–75S; discussion 89S–91S.

18 Moreno R, Waxman S, Rowe K, Verrier RL. Intrapericardial beta-adrenergic blockade with esmolol exerts a potent antitachycardic effect without depressing contractility. *J Cardiovasc Pharmacol* 2000; **36**: 722–7.

19 Ayers GM, Rho TH, Ben-David J, Besch HR Jr, Zipes DP. Amiodarone instilled into the canine pericardial sac migrates transmurally to produce electrophysiologic effects and suppress atrial fibrillation. *J Cardiovasc Electrophysiol* 1996; **7**: 713–21.

20 Labhasetwar V, Strickberger SA, Underwood T, Davis J, Levy RJ. Prevention of acute inducible atrial flutter in dogs by using an ibutilide-polymer-coated pacing electrode. *J Cardiovasc Pharmacol* 1998; **31**: 449–55.

21 Dorward PK, Flaim M, Ludbrook J. Blockade of cardiac nerves by intrapericardial local anaesthetics in the conscious rabbit. *Aust J Exp Biol Med Sci* 1983; **61**: 219–30.

22 Gleason JD, Nguyen KP, Wellenius GA, Kirkham JC, Verrier RL. Intrapericardial procaine produces marked and prolong reduction in vulnerability to vagally mediated atrial fibrillation. *Pacing Clin Electrophysiol* 2001; **24**: 600.

23 Ujhelyi MR, Sims JJ, Miller AW. Induction of electrical heterogeneity impairs ventricular defibrillation: an effect specific to regional conduction velocity slowing. *Circulation* 1999; **100**: 2534–40.

24 Sims JJ, Miller AW, Ujhelyi M. Myocardial vulnerability to ventricular fibrillation is regulated by dispersion in conduction, but not dispersion refractoriness. *Crit Care Med* 1999; **27**: A84.

25 Ujhelyi M, Hadsell K. Ibutilide is less proarrhythmic when instilled into the pericardial fluid space. *Pharmacotherapy* 2002; **22**: 1328.

26 Waxman S, Moreno R, Rowe KA, Verrier RL. Persistent primary coronary dilation induced by transatrial delivery of nitroglycerin into the pericardial space: a novel approach for local cardiac drug delivery. *J Am Coll Cardiol* 1999; **33**: 2073–7.

27 Matsunaga T, Warltier DC, Weihrauch DW *et al.* Ischemia-induced coronary collateral growth is dependent on vascular endothelial growth factor and nitric oxide. *Circulation* 2000; **102**: 3098–103.

28 Willerson JT, Igo SR, Yao SK *et al.* Localized administration of sodium nitroprusside enhances its protection against platelet aggregation in stenosed and injured coronary arteries. *Tex Heart Inst J* 1996; **23**: 1–8.

29 Fei L, Baron AD, Henry DP, Zipes DP. Intrapericardial delivery of L-arginine reduces the increased severity of ventricular arrhythmias during sympathetic stimulation in dogs with acute coronary occlusion: nitric oxide modulates sympathetic effects on ventricular electrophysiological properties. *Circulation* 1997; **96**: 4044–9.

30 Baek SH, Hrabie JA, Keefer LK *et al.* Augmentation of intrapericardial nitric oxide level by a prolonged-release nitric oxide donor reduces luminal narrowing after porcine coronary angioplasty. *Circulation* 2002; **105**: 2779–84.

31 Li D, Shinagawa K, Pang L *et al.* Effects of angiotensin-converting enzyme inhibition on development of the atrial fibrillation substrate in dogs with ventricular tachypacing-induced heart failure. *Circulation* 2001; **104**: 2608–14.

32 Hou D, Rogers PI, Toleikis PM, Hunter W, March KL. Intrapericardial paclitaxel delivery inhibits neointimal proliferation and promotes arterial enlargement after porcine coronary overstretch. *Circulation* 2000; **102**: 1575–81.

33 Hoit BD. Matrix metalloproteinases and atrial structural remodeling. *J Am Coll Cardiol* 2003; **42**: 345–7.

34 Lazarous DF, Shou M, Stiber JA *et al.* Adenoviral-mediated gene transfer induces sustained pericardial VEGF expression in dogs: effect on myocardial angiogenesis. *Cardiovasc Res* 1999; **44**: 294–302.

CHAPTER 14

Gene Therapy

J. Kevin Donahue, Amy D. McDonald, Heather Fraser,
Jeffrey J. Rade, Julie M. Miller, Alan H. Heldman

In concept, cardiac gene therapy has the potential to dramatically alter clinical practice. Whether by the modulation of existing gene expression or the introduction of new genes, if successfully developed it is not unreasonable to anticipate benefit for a number of congenital or acquired ailments. Despite significant forward momentum, serious obstacles remain which at present prevent wide application of gene therapy. In this chapter, we will review the core techniques of cardiac gene therapy, detail our own experience with atrioventricular (AV) node-targeted gene therapy, review the state of cellular genomic alteration towards automaticity (biological pacemaker), and summarize keys to further development.

Myocardial gene transfer techniques

Simply considered, the delivery of genetic material to the myocardium can be accomplished by several routes: (i) direct epicardium-based application; (ii) direct endocardium-based application; and (iii) transvascular application.

Epicardium-based gene transfer was first reported by Lamping and colleagues [1]. They injected a liquid vehicle containing an adenovirus into the pericardial space. They subsequently found that virus was unable to penetrate beyond the epimyocardial region. The addition of tetracycline to the vehicle caused an epicardial inflammatory reaction, which was associated with penetration deeper into the myocardial wall. However, transmural viral penetration was not achievable.

Direct injection into the myocardial wall using either epicardial or endocardial approaches has been reported. Lin and colleagues were the first to successfully demonstrate this technique [2], and Guzman and colleagues reported modifications which significantly increased its efficiency [3]. With injection, local delivery to an area within a few millimeters of the needle track can be achieved, but the lack of virus penetration beyond the local area prevents the use of this method for whole-organ applications. In addition, problems with inflammation and fibrosis in the injection region have been reported [3, 4]. This may be in part virus-dependent [5].

Transvascular gene therapy is a particularly attractive concept because of the theoretical opportunity for gene delivery to a large solid-tissue territory

(A)

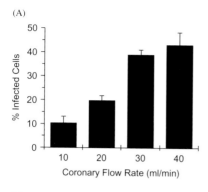

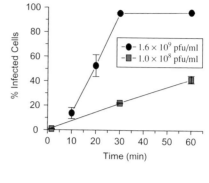

(B)

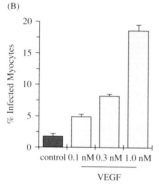

Fig. 14.1 Parameters that affect gene transfer efficiency. (A) Relationship between coronary flow rate, virus contact time and virus concentration obtained from intact rabbit hearts perfused using the Langendorff method. (Reprinted with permission from Donahue et al. *Proc Natl Acad Sci USA* 1997; **94**: 4664–8 [6].) (B) Improved gene transfer efficiency in the same model after increased microvascular permeability from exposure to vascular endothelial growth factor. (Reprinted with permission from Nagata et al. *J Mol Cell Cardiol* 2001; **33**: 575–80 [8].)

and the fact that percutaneous catheter-based techniques for transarterial or transvenous access and delivery are well established. However, there are significant issues with the efficiency of gene delivery, based primarily on difficulty in moving vector from the vascular space into myocardial tissue. We have shown that, for introduction via coronary arteries, blood flow rate, perfusion duration, and virus concentration in the perfusate each affects the magnitude of myocardial delivery (Fig. 14.1) [6]. A further increase in magnitude can be achieved by pretreating the conduit coronary artery with agents which increase microvascular permeability (Fig. 14.1) [7, 8]. Examples of such agents are serotonin, bradykinin, histamine, vascular endothelial growth factor, nitric oxide donors, phosphodiesterase inhibitors and cyclic GMP compounds. The transvascular delivery technique which we now use experimentally is a multistep process [9]. An orally administered phosphodiesterase inhibitor, sildenafil, is fed to the animals before the procedure. During the catheterization, the target artery is selectively cannulated. Over a period of several minutes, nitroglycerin and vascular endothelial growth factor are infused prior to the virus-containing solution. The solution is then infused rapidly as a single bolus and the catheter is removed. In a porcine model, this technique results in excellent myocardial gene transfer [9].

Atrioventricular node-targeted gene therapy

As has been detailed in foregoing chapters, ventricular rate control is a highly effective means of symptom management in atrial fibrillation patients [10, 11]. At present, means to achieve ventricular rate control include enteral pharmacotherapy (e.g. β and calcium channel blocking agents) and AV node ablation. However, pharmacotherapy is limited by inefficacy and intolerance, particularly in the elderly demographic which dominates atrial fibrillation. As discussed in detail in Chapter 6, AV node ablation is also limited by procedural risk and subsequent pacemaker-dependence. We hypothesized that AV node-targeted gene therapy could be used to achieve ventricular rate control without these limitations.

Our efforts thus far have been limited to a healthy porcine model in which atrial fibrillation was induced acutely by pacing [9]. We used first-generation adenovirus vectors. We hypothesized that amplification of the G-protein inhibitory α subunit ($G\alpha_{i2}$) would suppress adenylate cyclase activity, cyclic AMP production and calcium channel phosphorylation, and ultimately decrease AV nodal conduction (Fig. 14.2). Gene transfer was performed using the multistep transvascular technique detailed above. Selective cannulation of the AV nodal artery was accomplished percutaneously using a small diameter catheter which was occlusive. The solution containing the vector was delivered over 30 seconds, after which the catheter was removed. This technique achieves gene transfer to slightly less than half of the cells in the AV node, and results in a 6-fold increase in expression of the $G\alpha_{i2}$ protein (Fig. 14.3) [9]. At baseline (prior to gene transfer procedure) and 7 days after the procedure the ventricular rate during atrial fibrillation was assessed. We waited 7 days to permit production of the $G\alpha_{i2}$ protein; during this period animals were observed closely for the development of atrioventricular conduction abnormalities. Figure 14.4 compares ventricular rate control in animals receiving the $G\alpha_{i2}$ with control animals that received an inactive gene (β-galactosidase). During sinus rhythm,

G Protein Signaling Cascade

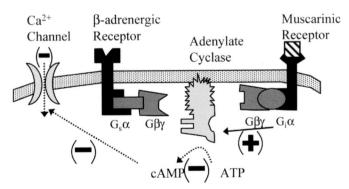

Fig. 14.2 Schematic of G-protein function in the AV node.

(a)

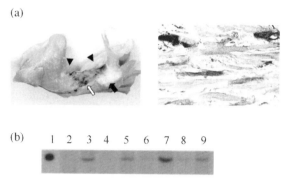

(b)

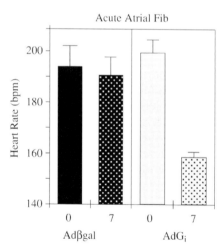

Fig. 14.3 *In vivo* gene transfer to the porcine atrioventricular node after pretreatment with nitroglycerin, vascular endothelial growth factor and sildenafil and perfusion with 7.5×10^{10} p.f.u. of an adenovirus encoding either β-galactosidase or the inhibitory G protein alpha subunit $G\alpha_{i2}$. (A) Gross and microscopic views of the AV node after staining for β-galactosidase activity. For details of delivery method see reference 9. (B) Western blot from AV nodal tissue probed for $G\alpha_{i2}$. (Reprinted with permission from Donahue *et al. Nat Med* 2000; **6**: 1395–8 [9].)

Fig. 14.4 Ventricular rate during acutely induced atrial fibrillation in sedated pigs. For details see reference 9. (Reprinted with permission from Donahue *et al. Nat Med* 2000; **6**: 1395–8 [9].)

members of the $G\alpha_{i2}$ group evidenced slowing of AV conduction and increased refractoriness. Spontaneous second- or third-degree AV block was not observed, nor was there evidence of tachyproarrhythmia or alteration in mechanical structure and function. During atrial fibrillation, the ventricular rate in the β-galactosidase group was unchanged relative to baseline. In contrast, in the $G\alpha_{i2}$ group the ventricular rate was approximately 20% lower than at baseline. This observation persisted during adrenergic stimulation.

Based on these data, we believe that targeted AV nodal gene transfer may be a viable method for ventricular rate control during atrial fibrillation. Our eventual plan is to evaluate this technique in a clinical trial.

Biological pacemaker

We define the term 'biological pacemaker' as any technique which uses intrinsic or exogenously introduced organic matter to promote cardiac automaticity. In this quest, two broad approaches have been used thus far. The first involves cell therapy, in which exogenous cells with automatic properties are transplanted in their native state or after modification. The state of this art is reviewed in Chapter 15. The other approach has been to modify the gene component of intrinsic cardiac cells to promote automaticity. To this end three different strategies have been pursued [12]: (i) upregulation of the effects of adrenergic drive on automaticity; (ii) reduction of outward (repolarizing) current; and (iii) increasing inward current during diastole.

Upregulation of the effects of adrenergic drive on automaticity

Edelberg and colleagues injected a plasmid containing the gene encoding the β_2-adrenergic receptor into the atria of animals [13, 14]. They reasoned that atrial cells which were successfully transfected would manifest increased responsiveness to endogenous or administered adrenergic agonists, engendering an increased heart rate. This goal was realized, but was short-lived.

Reduction of outward (repolarizing) current

This tends to suppress spontaneous depolarization. Miake and colleagues used an adenoviral vector to transfect guinea-pig ventricular myocytes *in vivo* with an altered gene encoding one of the pore-forming unit proteins of a potassium channel (Kir2.1), which when incorporated into the channel caused suppression of channel (I_{K1}) function [15]. In these animals, ectopic ventricular rhythms were observed to occur spontaneously, and phase 4 depolarization was documented in the isolated myocytes studied *in vitro*.

Increasing inward current during diastole

Towards this goal, Qu and colleagues transfected rat ventricular myocytes in culture and *in vivo* with a gene construct which increased the activity of I_f, an inward depolarizing current which is the primary pacemaker current of the heart [16, 17]. In cell culture, a significantly greater beating rate was seen in the transfected myocytes than in controls. In animals, spontaneous automaticity was achieved in the injected zones (atrium and ventricle). This group has also demonstrated the feasibility of transplanting mesenchymal stem cells, in which I_f is enhanced by prior transfection, into live animal hearts [18]. In these animals, spontaneous automaticity emanating from injected regions was observed, and immunohistological analysis documented the presence of viable transplanted stems cells forming gap junctions with host myocytes. These data suggest that stem cells could function as a delivery vehicle for genetically modified cells with specific functionality. The use of cell transplantation towards pacemaker reconstitution is discussed in detail in Chapter 15.

Keys to development

We believe that our experience with AV nodal gene transfer and that with pacemaker reconstitution illustrate the promise of cardiac gene therapy. However, there are serious problems which must be overcome if gene therapy is to become important clinically. First, previous reports have demonstrated poor long-term gene expression with current viral vectors [4]. Loss of gene expression appears to be in part related to immune-mediated inflammation. Adenoviruses are notoriously immunogenic, for reasons that are unclear. Preliminary reports using adenovirus vectors from which all viral genes have been deleted have suggested the possibility of long-term expression, but these data have been inconsistent. Recently, it has become apparent that adeno-associated virus (AAV) vectors appear to be less immunogenic and to be associated with persistence of expression of transferred genes [19]. It is possible that this is related to the fact that AAV does not encode viral proteins, but specific mechanisms are as yet unclear. Experience with AAV vectors for cardiac use is as yet nascent. Secondly, even with targeted introduction to the heart, such as by injection or subselective perfusion, transfer is also manifest in other organs. For example, in our experience with transvascular AV node-targeted transfer, low-level expression of the $G\alpha_{i2}$ gene product was detected in liver, ovary and kidney [9]. Similar findings have been reported after direct intramyocardial injection [20]. Although studies to date have not demonstrated toxicity of this collateral expression *per se*, it is clear that this phenomenon will need to be thoroughly vetted with regard to the specific gene product and dose planned for any human application. Evolution of gene therapy is likely to include methods for increasing tissue specificity by molecular alteration of the apparatus that the virus uses to attach to the host cell [21]. Cardiac application of this technique has not yet been reported, and it will require improved insight into the molecular fingerprint of the myocyte surface and mechanisms by which viruses attach and penetrate.

Acknowledgments

The authors would like to acknowledge and thank Dr Eduardo Marbán for advice and mentorship, the National Institutes of Health, NHLBI section, the American Heart Association, and the Deutschen Forschungsgemeinschaft for research funding support, and St Jude Medical Corporation for donation of the pacemakers mentioned in this chapter.

References

1 Lamping K, Rios CD, Chun JA *et al*. Intrapericardial administration of adenovirus for gene transfer. *Am J Physiol* 1997; **272**: H310–17.
2 Lin H, Parmacek M, Morle G, Bolling S, Leiden J. Expression of recombinant genes in the myocardium in vivo after direct injection of DNA. *Circulation* 1990; **82**: 2217–21.

3 Guzman RJ, Lemarchand P, Crystal R, Epstein SE, Finkel T. Efficient gene transfer into myocardium by direct injection of adenovirus vectors. *Circ Res* 1993; **73**: 1202−7.

4 Wright M, Wightman L, Lilley C *et al.* In vivo myocardial gene transfer: optimization, evaluation and direct comparison of gene transfer vectors. *Basic Res Cardiol* 2001; **96**: 227−36.

5 Kaplitt M, Xiao X, Samulski R *et al.* Long term gene transfer in porcine myocardium after coronary infusion of an adeno-associated virus vector. *Ann Thorac Surg* 1996; **62**: 1669−76.

6 Donahue J, Kikkawa K, Johns D, Marban E, Lawrence J. Ultrarapid, highly efficient viral gene transfer to the heart. *Proc Natl Acad Sci USA* 1997; **94**: 4664−8.

7 Donahue J, Kikkawa K, Thomas AD, Marban E, Lawrence J. Acceleration of widespread adenoviral gene transfer to intact rabbit hearts by coronary perfusion with low calcium and serotonin. *Gene Ther* 1998; **5**: 630−4.

8 Nagata K, Marban E, Lawrence J, Donahue J. Phosphodiesterase inhibitor-mediated potentiation of adenovirus delivery to myocardium. *J Mol Cell Cardiol* 2001; **33**: 575−80.

9 Donahue J, Heldman A, Fraser H *et al.* Focal modification of electrical conduction in the heart by viral gene transfer. *Nat Med* 2000; **6**: 1395−8.

10 Wyse D, Waldo A, DiMarco J *et al.* A comparison of rate control and rhythm control in patients with atrial fibrillation. *N Engl J Med* 2002; **347**: 1825−33.

11 Van Gelder I, Hagens V, Bosker H *et al.* A comparison of rate control and rhythm control in patients with recurrent persistent atrial fibrillation. *N Engl J Med* 2002; **347**: 1834−40.

12 Rosen MR, Brink PR, Cohen IS, Robinson RB. Cardiac pacemakers for the new millennium. *Hellenic J Cardiol* 2004; **45**: 205−7.

13 Edelberg JM, Aird WC, Rosenberg RD. Enhancement of murine cardiac chronotropy by the molecular transfer of the human β_2-adrenergic receptor cDNA. *J Clin Invest* 1998; **101**: 337−43.

14 Edelberg JM, Huang DT, Josephson ME, Rosenberg RD. Molecular enhancement of porcine cardiac chronotropy. *Heart* 2001; **86**: 559−62.

15 Miake J, Marban E, Nuss HB. Gene therapy: biological pacemaker created by gene transfer. *Nature* 2002; **419**: 132−3.

16 Qu J, Plotnikov AN, Danilo P Jr *et al.* Expression and function of a biological pacemaker in canine heart. *Circulation* 2003; **107**: 1106−9.

17 Plotnikov AN, Sisunov EA, Qu J *et al.* Biological pacemaker implanted in canine left bundle branch provides ventricular escape rhythms that have physiologically acceptable rates. *Circulation* 2004; **109**: 506−12.

18 Potapova I, Plotnikov A, Lu Z *et al.* Human mesenchymal stem cells as a gene delivery system to create cardiac pacemakers. *Circ Res* 2004; **94**: 952−9.

19 Mount J, Herzog R, Tillson D *et al.* Sustained phenotypic correction of hemophilia B dogs with a factor IX null mutation by liver-directed gene therapy. *Blood* 2002; **99**: 2670−6.

20 Kass-Eisler A, Falck-Pedersen E, Elfenbein DH *et al.* The impact of developmental stage, route of administration and the immune system on adenovirus-mediated gene transfer. *Gene Ther* 1994; **1**: 395−402.

21 Curiel D. Strategies to adapt adenoviral vectors for targeted delivery. *Ann NY Acad Sci* 1999; **886**: 158−71.

CHAPTER 15

Tissue Engineering

Randall J. Lee

The clinical goals of tissue engineering are to restore, repair, or replace damaged or lost tissues in the body [1]. Cardiac tissue engineering is a rapidly developing field [2]. Key fronts in the developmental effort are cell transplantation and biological scaffolding. For example, recent reports have demonstrated that skeletal myoblasts, when transplanted into a cardiac milieu, survive and form contractile myofibers in normal and injured myocardium [3, 4]. Autologous stem cells have also been shown to improve left ventricular function following a myocardial infarction [5]. Introduction of cell scaffolds, even in the absence of transplanted cells, has also shown promise [6]. Combinations of scaffolds and transplanted cells are being assessed.

Not surprisingly, the primary foci of cardiac tissue engineering have been the improvement of left ventricular mechanical dysfunction and/or amelioration of the ischemic burden. As regards arrhythmia, it is possible that progress in this area will have tangential benefit. However, cardiac tissue engineering with the primary intent of treatment of bradyarrhythmias or tachyarrhythmias may also be feasible. Development in this area may include methods for promoting automaticity and conduction, as well as achieving insulation; these are discussed below. If successful, we believe that development may eventually yield therapeutic applications for patients with atrial fibrillation.

Biological pacemaker

We define the term 'biological pacemaker' to mean any technique which uses intrinsic or exogenously introduced organic matter to provide automaticity. In the previous chapter, gene therapy techniques toward this goal were reviewed, in which existing cardiac cells are coaxed into genomic modification so as to alter their electrophysiological properties in favor of automaticity. In this section, I examine transplantation into the heart of exogenous cells or other materials.

In the how-to of reconstituting a pacemaker, one can consider several cell sources. Conceptually, the simplest choice is autologous transplantation of atrial cells, which prominently manifest the inward depolarizing current I_f, which is the primary pacemaker current of the heart [7]. Clinical sinus node dysfunction does not appear to be due primarily to abnormalities in I_f. Thus, in theory one could obtain tissue from the sinus node region, select and amplify cells expressing I_f *ex vivo*, and reinject them into the same or other regions. Certainly, imaging and catheter technologies are currently available to achieve targeted intramyocardial introduction, whether endocardially or epicardially based. In support of the feasibility of this approach, a report by Ruhparwar and colleagues detailed the implantation of fetal cardiac myocytes (including sinus node cells) into the left ventricle. Histological studies showed survival of grafted cells, formation of gap junctions between donor and recipient cells, and spontaneous generation of QRS complexes with a morphology consistent with formation in the implanted cell region [8]. Towards clinical application, a key hurdle will be amplification of mature pacemaker cells. Gepstein and colleagues have provided preliminary data to suggest that subpopulations of embryonic stem cells initiate impulses in a fashion similar to mature pacemaker cells [9]. Whether impulse generation is based on I_f is not known. It is important to note that although I_f is a prominent current which distinguishes pacemaker cells, the number and choreography of gene products which yield phase 4 depolarization is not yet clear.

A second potential cell source for pacemaker reconstitution is autologous cells without intrinsic pacemaker function. Examples would include skeletal myoblasts or skin fibroblasts. These cells have been used in humans. These cells are attractive because of their autologous origin, high proliferative potential *in vitro*, advanced stage of differentiation (myogenic restricted lineage commitment, which virtually eliminates the risk of tumorigenicity) and resistance to ischemic damage [10]. Given their lack of pacemaker activity, these cells would need to be re-engineered; as mentioned above and detailed in the Chapter 14, one promising method for this would be genomic modification. It is not clear that these cells, even if directly introduced to the anatomical sinus node, would intercalate and become functioning members. Ominous in this regard is the experience with these cells in animal models (primarily introduction into the left ventricle after acute myocardial infarction) which demonstrates lack of electrical coupling between engrafted and host cardiomyocytes [11]. Sinus node anatomy is not discrete; it is rather complex, diffuse and multidimensional, comprising both cardiomyocytes and support cells [12]. It is unclear how important this anatomy is for normal pacemaker function. Of course, one need not by necessity conceptualize the reconstitution of pacemaker function at the anatomical site of the sinus node. However, it is worth remembering that the sinus node derives its functionality not only from intrinsic properties but also from extrinsic influences. For example, as emphasized in a previous chapter, one key element of the healthy sinus node is robust interaction with neural forces, both vagal and adrenergic. A pathological interaction can actually promote arrhythmia. Whether exogenously introduced cells would interact healthfully with the nervous system is unknown.

A third potential cell class for pacemaker reconstitution is the adult-derived stem cell. It is possible that each organ has stem cells. That cardiac stem cells actually exist was first suggested after demonstration of replicating cells in the adult heart in pathological states [13]. Two potential sources of cardiac stem cells have been suggested: (i) the bone marrow, from which they are released and engraft in the heart, either as a low-level process of ongoing renewal or in response to injury; (ii) the local cell population. Given the still elusive nature of the cardiac stem cell, the most common derivations of adult-derived stem cells have been bone marrow-derived stem cells (BMSC), mesenchymal stem cells and endothelial progenitor cells. Adult stem cells, like myoblasts (discussed above), have the advantage of autologous origin. However, unlike myoblasts they possess plasticity, theoretically allowing them to change their phenotype in response to influences such as organ-environment cues. Although it is possible that this property will be beneficial, it may also produce complications (e.g. tumorigenicity). BMSC have been used in humans in preliminary studies, which as mentioned above were geared primarily to improvement in the mechanics and/or amelioration of ischemia. A bone marrow aspirate comprises many different cell types, the individual characteristics of which are incompletely characterized. In fact, at present the identification of multipotent BMSC is a developing science, and which of these cells may be suited to cardiac applications is unknown. Thus far, it appears that the *ex vivo* amplification of known stem cells is technically challenging, as is the *in vivo* mobilization of these cells (e.g. with a drug such as 5-azacytidine [14]). For a number of reasons, clinical studies have thus far used unfractionated marrow (mononuclear cells), with mixed results [10]. Most of the favorable data appear to point to a more important role for these cells in promoting angiogenesis than in cardiomyocyte regeneration. In fact, there is controversy as to whether the BMSC used are even capable of transdifferentiation into cardiomyocytes [10]. In terms of conceptualizing use for pacemaker reconstruction, in addition to the above, as for myoblasts these cells would need to be re-engineered in the direction of spontaneous automaticity. A promising finding has been the suggestion of coupling between host cells and graft cells via connexins [15]. A recent report by Potapova and colleagues demonstrated the feasibility of transplanting mesenchymal stem cells, in which the primary depolarizing (pacemaker) current (I_f) was enhanced by genomic alteration, into live animal hearts [16]. In these animals, spontaneous automaticity emanating from injected regions was observed, and immuno-histological analysis documented the presence of viable transplanted stems cells forming gap junctions with host myocytes. These data suggest that stem cells could function as a delivery vehicle for genetically modified cells with specific functionality, and indicate that the line of demarcation between gene therapy and cell therapy (see also Chapter 14) is becoming progressively blurred. Interestingly, rather than viral transfection, these investigators used a technique called electroporation to achieve the desired genomic alteration of the stem cells. This process may bypass some of the concerns regarding collateral risk (e.g. tumorigenicity) in the use of virally transfected cells. Finally, a continuing problem with BMSC, one common to all exogenous cells, is cell death. Thus far, this appears to encompass the vast majority of cells introduced in various models. It is probably due to multiple mechanisms, including physical trauma associated with introduction, inflammation, apoptosis and ischemia.

A fourth potential cell class for pacemaker reconstitution is the embryonic stem cell (ESC). ESC are pluripotent cells derived from the inner cell mass of non-used blastocysts (preimplantation embryos), or blastocysts created for therapeutic applications by nuclear transfer [17, 18]. These cells are characterized by their capacity to proliferate in an undifferentiated state for a prolonged period in culture. Afterwards, they can differentiate into every tissue type in the body. Previous studies have demonstrated that ESC can differentiate into cardiomyocytes, including those with specialized electrophysiological properties [19–25], and can form stable intracardiac grafts [26]. Key hurdles to their clinical use include durability, proarrhythmia and tumorigenicity.

Finally, an acellular material with potential for pacemaker reconstitution is extracellular matrix material (ECM). ECM is the connective tissue scaffolding into which cells are seeded to form a functional organ. Regardless of the organ, ECM is geometrically and biochemically complex [6]. Preliminary evaluation of ECM in cardiac application has been promising, demonstrating repopulation of damaged regions with viable cardiomyocytes [6]. It is possible that ECM acts as a multidimensional 'road map,' which is recognized by regional myocyte precursors but is usually absent after damage. It is more likely that the biochemical composition of the ECM material (chemoattractant factors, growth factors, etc.) promotes tissue regeneration. In this regard, exogenous cell therapies and ECM may have something in common. As with ECM, it is possible that any beneficial effect of cell therapy is not the cell *per se* (e.g. the cells or their successors do not persist) but rather the scaffolding (physical, biochemical, etc.) presented to the region that induces tissue regeneration. As for pacemaker reconstitution, a role for ECM is conjectural at this time.

In summary, the art of transplantation of exogenous cells and acellular material to reconstitute pacemaker function is largely hypothetical. To move towards clinical relevance, many scientific and technical issues will need to be addressed, prominent among which are functionality, durability, immunogenicity, arrhythmogenicity and tumorigenicity. In addition, logistical, ethical and religious concerns may arise, revolving around cell sourcing and transplantation procedures.

Biological conductor

The intercellular electromechanical coupling of cardiomyocyte is a core requirement for normal heart function. Cardiomyocytes are coupled by intercalated disks consisting of junctions. Connexins are the major gap junction proteins and they differ in their specific structure according to the myocardial region [27, 28]. Overexpression of connexin has been suggested as a means to enhance intracardiac cardiac conduction [29]. We recently characterized the transduction of skeletal myoblasts by a retroviral vector expressing the connexin 43 gene [30]. The transduced cells were injected into the atrioventricular (AV) node of immunodeficient rats and found to improve conduction through the AV node compared with those which were injected with non-transduced cells. Given that conduction delay and blocking are key elements of the atrial fibrillation substrate, it is tempting to speculate that atrial cell transplantation to achieve a global effect of overexpression of connexins would result in improved conduction and resistance to arrhythmia. Means by which such transplantation might be achieved are as yet unknown. Of course, heterogeneous delivery might actually be proarrhythmic.

Biological insulator

As discussed in earlier chapters, atrial ablation is a developing strategy for the suppression of atrial fibrillation. The core functional element of ablation is conduction block which is limited and strategically located so as to interfere with the initiation and/or sustenance of activation wavelets. In addition to necessitating the destruction of otherwise functional tissue, the act of ablation carries risks, which, in addition to access, include collateral damage (cardiac and non-cardiac) and cardioembolism. In addition, after ablation there appears to be a significant risk of tissue recovery, and this phenomenon probably contributes to clinical inefficacy. For these reasons, it is reasonable to consider other means by which regional conduction block may be achieved.

Using cardiomyocytes from fetal, neonatal or adult rats, Reinecke and colleagues observed that grafted tissue is usually separated from host tissue by collagenous scar [31]. It is likely that this region would have resisted traversal by electrical activation. It is also likely that the cellular electrophysiological properties of the grafted material might evolve so as to promote conduction block. For example, we examined the electrophysiological properties of skeletal myoblasts and myotubes (multinucleated cells to which myoblasts may differentiate) *in vitro*. Skeletal myoblasts were isolated by enzymatic dispersion from the hind limb muscle of 2- to 5-day-old neonatal rats. Myoblasts differentiated into multinucleated myotubes when the growth medium was replaced with differential medium. Myoblasts and myotubes incubated for between 2 and 14 days were studied. The whole-cell configuration of the patch-clamp technique was used to record action potentials. Measurements included resting membrane potential (RMP), action potential amplitude (APA), action potential upstroke velocity (V_{max}), and action potential duration at 50% repolarization (APD_{50}; Fig. 15.1). There was no significant difference in RMP between days 8 and 10–14. The APA increased and reached a peak value at 10–11 days, then decreased in parallel until a nadir at 13–14 days. Changes in V_{max} paralleled APA. Finally, the minimum APD_{50} value occurred at 11–12 days and then increased. These data highlight the relative electrical inexcitability of myoblasts before 7 days. Additionally, the data confirm that skeletal myoblasts and myotubes have short action potentials. This corroborates computer modeling experiments which predict that tight coupling is necessary for myocardial cells to excite skeletal myoblasts/myotubes [32]. We further assessed the electrophysiological consequences of skeletal muscle transplantation into the myocardium using a whole-animal (rat) model of AV node injection. Changes

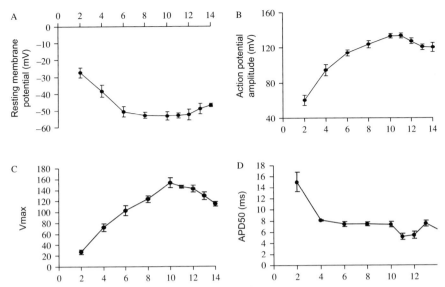

Fig. 15.1 Changes in action potential parameters during different periods after skeletal myoblast isolation (see also text). (A) Resting membrane potential. (B) Action potential amplitude. (C) Maximum action potential upstroke velocity. (D) Action potential duration demarcating 50% repolarization.

in AV node function after injection provide an accessible window for judging the effect of the injection. A single injection of skeletal myoblasts (1×10^5 cells in 15 μl) was used. As opposed to a control injected group (acellular vehicle), significant changes were observed in the AV nodal function indices of the myoblast injection group, including Wenkebach cycle length (70.0 ± 4.4 versus 57.0 ± 5.0 ms) and AV nodal refractory period (113.8 ± 5.6 versus 87.0 ± 6.2 ms). Interestingly, histological examination of the AV nodes of the myoblast injection group revealed that, on average, only approximately 10% of the node territory was involved with myoblasts, and there was minimal inflammation. Histologically, the AV conduction axis appeared normal in control vehicle injections. These data lend credence to the concept that certain cell therapies can produce conduction slowing or block independent of inflammation or fibrosis, presumably as a result of a reduction in the aggregate excitability of the cellular syncytium in the altered region.

Another cell source which may be worthy of consideration for the purpose of promoting insulation is fibroblasts. Fibroblasts have reproducible cellular electrophysiological properties. They are readily available, easy to culture and relatively resistant to hypoxia. In an ischemia–reperfusion model of myocardial injury, fibroblasts were shown to significantly decrease the induction of ventricular tachyarrhythmias and significantly increase the ventricular fibrillation thresholds. Additionally, in a porcine model of acute myocardial infarction, autologous fibroblasts transplanted into the infarct area resulted in a decrease in ventricular ectopy without any proarrhythmic events. It is reasonable to hypothesize that the amelioration of arrhythmia burden observed in each of these studies was due to the insulating influence of the transplanted cells, reducing the likelihood of re-entry. Having said this, it is important to note that the promotion of conduction block, although of potential interest in therapy for atrial fibrillation, is probably one of the elements underlying what appears to be a *proarrhythmic* effect observed during some clinical trials of ventricular cell therapy [10]. Obviously, if tissue-engineered changes in conduction are to become clinically useful, key elements will have to be understood. As can be gleaned from the foregoing, prominent among these will be insight into the host response to graft introduction, graft dosing, and the durability of the effect.

References

1 Levenberg S, Langer R. Advances in tissue engineering. *Curr Top Dev Biol* 2004; **61**: 113–34.

2 Weisel RD. Cardiac restoration by cell transplantation. *Int J Cardiol* 2004; **95** (Suppl. 1): S5–7.

3 Weisel RD, Li RK, Mickle DA, Yau TM. Cell transplantation comes of age. *J Thorac Cardiovasc Surg* 2001; **121**: 835–6.

4 Murry C, Wiseman RW, Schwartz SM, Hauschka SD. Skeletal myoblast transplantation for repair of myocardial necrosis. *J Clin Invest* 1996; **98**: 2512–23.

5 Liu J, Hu O, Wang Z *et al.* Autologous stem cell transplantation for myocardial repair. *Am J Physiol* 2004; **287**: H501–11.

6 Badylak S, Obermiller J, Geddes L, Matheny R. Extracellular matrix for myocardial repair. *Heart Surg Forum* 2003; **6**: E20–6.

7 Di Francesco D. A study of the ionic nature of the pacemaker current in calf purkinje fibres. *J Physiol* 1981; **314**: 377–93.

8 Ruhparwar A, Tebbenjohans J, Niehaus M *et al.* Transplanted fetal cardiomyocytes as cardiac pacemaker. *Eur J Cardiothorac Surg* 2002; **21**: 853–7.

9 Gepstein L. Derivation and potential applications of human embryonic stems cells. *Circ Res* 2002; **91**: 866–76.

10 Menasche P. Cellular transplantation: hurdles remaining before widespread clinical use. *Curr Opin Cardiol* 2004; **19**: 154–61.

11 Dowell JD, Rubart M, Pasumarthi KBS, Soonpaa MH, Field LJ. Myocyte and myogenic stem cell transplantation in the heart. *Cardiovasc Res* 2003; **58**: 336–50.

12 Boineau JP, Canavan TE, Schuessler RB *et al.* Demonstration of a widely distributed atrial pacemaker complex in the human heart. *Circulation* 1988; **77**: 1221–37.

13 Beltrami AP, Urbanek K, Kajstura J *et al.* Evidence that human cardiac myocytes divide after myocardial infarction. *N Engl J Med* 2001; **344**: 1750–5.

14 Bittira B, Kuang JQ, Al-Khaldi A, Shum-Tim D, Chiu RCJ. In vitro preprogramming of marrow stromal cells for myocardial regeneration. *Ann Thorac Surg* 2002; **74**: 1154–60.

15 Orlic D, Kajstura J, Chimenti S *et al.* Bone marrow cells regenerate infarcted myocardium. *Nature* 2001; **410**: 701–5.

16 Potapova I, Plotnikov A, Lu Z *et al.* Human mesenchymal stem cells as a gene delivery system to create cardiac pacemakers. *Circ Res* 2004; **94**: 952–9.

17 Evans M, Kaufman MH. Establishment in culture of pluripotential cells from mouse embryos. *Nature* 1981; **292**: 154–6.

18 Bongso T, Fong CY, Ng SC, Ratnam SS. Isolation and culture of inner cell mass cells from human blastocysts. *Hum Reprod* 1994; **9**: 2110–17.

19 Sanchez A, Jones WK, Bulick J, Doetschman T, Robbins J. Myosin heavy chain gene expression in mouse embryoid bodies: an in vitro developmental study. *J Biol Chem* 1991; **226**: 22419–26.

20 Miller-Hance W, LaCorbiere M, Fuller SJ *et al*. In vitro chamber specification during embryonic stem cell cardiogenesis. Expression of the ventricular myosin light chain-2 gene is independent of heart tube formation. *J Biol Chem* 1993; **268**: 25244–52.

21 Muthuchamy M, Pajak L, Howles L, Doetschman T, Dieczorek DF. Developmental analysis of tropomyosin gene expression in embryonic stem cells and mouse embryos. *Mol Cell Biol* 1993; **13**: 3311–23.

22 Boer P. Activation of the gene for type-b natriuretic factor in mouse stem cell cultures induced from cardiac myogenesis. *Biochem Biophys Res Commun* 1994; **199**: 954–61.

23 Ganim J, Luo W, Ponniah S *et al*. Mouse phospholamban gene expression during development in vivo and in vitro. *Circ Res* 1992; **71**: 1021–30.

24 Metzger J, Lin WI, Samuelson LC. Transition in cardiac contractile sensitivity to calcium during the in vitro differentiation of mouse embryonic stem cells. *J Cell Biol* 1994; **126**: 701–11.

25 Maltsev V, Rohwedel J, Hescheler J, Wobus AM. Embryonic stem cells differentiate in vitro into cardiomyocytes representing sinus-nodal, atrial and ventricular cell types. *Mech Dev* 1993; **44**: 41–50.

26 Klug M, Soonpaa MH, Koh GY, Field LJ. Genetically selected cardiomyocytes from differentiating embryonic stem cells form stable intracardiac grafts. *J Clin Invest* 1996; **98**: 216–24.

27 Saffitz JE, Kanter HL, Green KG, Tolley TK, Beyer EC. Tissue-specific determinants of anisotropic conduction velocity in canine atrial and ventricular myocardium. *Circ Res* 1994; **74**: 1065–70.

28 Davis LM, Kanter HL, Beyer EC, Safitz JE. Distinct gap junction protein phenotypes in cardiac tissues with disparate conduction properties. *J Am Coll Cardiol* 1994; **24**: 1124–34.

29 Suzuki K, Brand NJ, Allen S *et al*. Overexpression of connexin 43 in skeletal myoblasts: relevance to cellular transplantation to the heart. *J Thorac Cardiovasc Surg* 2001; **122**: 759–66.

30 Lee RJ, Sievers RE, Gallinghouse GJ, Ursell PC. Development of a model of complete heart block in rates. *J Appl Physiol* 1998; **85**: 758–63.

31 Reinecke H, Ming Z, Bartosek T, Murry CE. Survival, integration and differentiation of cardiomyocyte grafts: a study in normal and injured rats. *Circulation* 1999; **100**: 193–202.

32 Shaw RM, Lee RJ. Requirements for transplanted skeletal cells to function electrically within ventricular myocardium. *J Am Coll Cardiol* 2002; **39**: 192A.

Index